Hyperbaric Oxygenation For Cerebral Palsy and the Brain-Injured Child

A Promising Treatment

Featuring HBO and Mitochondrial Cytopathies

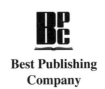

Best Publishing Company

Hyperbaric Oxygenation For Cerebral Palsy and the Brain-Injured Child

A Promising Treatment

Featuring HBO and Mitochondrial Cytopathies

Richard A. Neubauer, MD

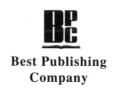

Best Publishing Company

Photo Credit: Barbara Gula

First Edition 2002
Second Edition 2005

Design: Jill McAdoo
            Rudy Ramos
            Rebecca Henestofel

Cover: U Hon Cheang

Editor: Jim Joiner
            Stephanie Karles
            Virginia Neubauer
            Barbara Zunich

ISBN: 0-941332-99-3
Library of Congress Catalog Number: 200111 7820

Best Publishing Company
website: www.bestpub.com
2355 North Steves Boulevard
P.O. Box 30100
Flagstaff, AZ 86003-0100 USA
Tele: 928.527.1055

Table of Contents

Dedication

This book is dedicated to Dr. Richard Neubauer, a pioneer in the field of hyperbaric oxygenation therapy for children with cerebral palsy and brain injuries.

Dr. Neubauer's vision of how HBOT might improve the lives of these children became his dream and his avocation. In spite of the many obstacles he had to overcome and the lack of support from the medical community, he maintained his belief in hyperbaric oxygenation therapy for these children. He steadfastly persisted to bring his ideas to completion.

Today, his dedicated work has made a significant impact on the way the medical community addresses children with CP and brain injuries, and his devotion to his belief is bringing benefits to potentially millions of CP and brain injured children, worldwide.

Dr. Neubauer, we salute you. Your dream has become a reality. This story of Rebecca proves how right you were.

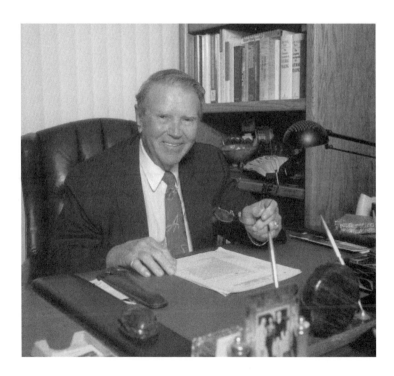

ABOUT THE AUTHOR

Richard A. Neubauer, M.D.

Dr. Richard Neubauer, Medical Director of the Ocean Hyperbaric Neurologic Center in Lauderdale-by-the-Sea, Florida, is internationally known and respected as a pioneer and leader in the field of hyperbaric medicine. He is a graduate of the University of Virginia Medical School, with a specialization in internal medicine, and was associated with Philadelphia General Hospital for many years. In this position he served as Chief of the Special Medical Ward and the Medical Renal Clinic as well as the Director of Medical Research for the Municipal Welfare Clinic. Prior to his keen interest in the developing field of hyperbaric medicine, Dr. Neubauer had a thriving internal medicine practice for more than ten years in Lauderdale-by-the-Sea. When he first began his practice in this small but growing community, he was the only internal medicine specialist.

As one of the leading proponents of hyperbaric oxygen therapy (HBOT), Dr. Neubauer has been using pressurized oxygen to treat patients with a variety of neurological disorders since 1972. He formed a partnership with Dr. Edgar End (co-inventor of the underwater breathing device known as the Aqualung and developer of the suits worn by "frogmen" in World War II), and much of their work centered around patients with acute and long-term stroke, brain injury, and coma. Dr. Neubauer also collaborated with Dr. Sheldon Gottlieb, former professor of biological sciences and physiology at the University of Southern Alabama, who helped to disseminate, scientifically evaluate, and validate Dr. Neubauer's original observations in the treatment of multiple sclerosis. Dr. Gottlieb later worked with Dr. Neubauer to pioneer a new technique of interventional brain imaging to ascertain the metabolic changes acheived with hyperbaric oxygen therapy in brain injury.

In time, Dr. Neubauer's primary focus became the use of hyperbaric oxygen to recover marginally damaged brain tissue. He gradually gave up his internal medicine practice and devoted his attention to the treatment of patients with acute and long-standing neurological defects from stroke, traumatic brain injury, anoxic encephalopathies, and diseases such as multiple sclerosis, Lyme disease, AIDS, reflex sympathetic dystrophy, and other cerebral vascular insufficiencies and related illnesses. As Dr. Neubauer worked with patients suffering from various types of neurological insults, he became fascinated with the potential of HBOT in treating cerebral palsy. By the late 1990s, this was one of the main foci of his practice. Dr. Neubauer has treated more than 400 children with cerebral palsy, and many of them have gained a better quality of life as a result of these treatments.

The Ocean Hyperbaric Neurologic Center is believed to be the original facility specializing in the neurologic applications of hyperbaric oxygenation and the potentially recoverable brain. Dr. Neubauer was one of the first doctors to use SPECT scanning with hyperbaric oxygenation to document changes in brain activity after HBO treatments. His center was also one of the first independent facilities in the United States to install its own gamma camera for digital imaging of brain function. In all, Dr. Neubauer has treated more than 2000 patients whose various diseases and neurological conditions have improved through the use of HBOT.

Dr. Neubauer is currently a member of the following organizations:
- International Society of Hyperbaric Medicine
- European Undersea and Baromedical Society
- Italian Hyperbaric Society
- Cuban Hyperbaric Society
- PanAmerican Hyperbaric Society
- American Medical Association
- Broward County Medical Association
- Florida Medical Association
- American Society of Internal Medicine
- American Association of Physicians and Surgeons
- Society of Nuclear Medicine
- American Academy of Neurology
- Florida Physicians Association

In addition to providing medical services and leadership to his clinic in Lauderdale-by-the-Sea, he is also on the active staff of Holy Cross and North Ridge General hospitals. Dr. Neubauer served as founding President and CEO of the American College of Hyperbaric Medicine, President of the Gulf Coast chapter of the Undersea and Hyperbaric Medical Society, Founding Member and Board Chairman of the National Alliance of Physicians and Surgeons, and is a Fellow in the Royal Society of Medicine. He has been honored and recognized by many associations and countries for his work in hyperbaric medicine and his leadership for advances in hyperbaric oxygen therapy, and has been proposed for nomination for the Nobel Prize in Medicine.

Interest in the field of HBOT is growing rapidly, both within the United States and internationally, and Dr. Neubauer travels to various conferences and symposiums around the world to educate both the medical community and the lay public on the uses of hyperbaric oxygen therapy. He has made presentations on the subject of HBOT in more than 15 different countries, including Cuba, France, Greece, Switzerland, Germany, Denmark, Japan, and Israel. In addition, Dr. Neubauer is the author of more than 45 published papers on the use of hyperbaric oxygen therapy and SPECT scans, and is the co-author of the book *Hyperbaric Oxygen Therapy*. Dr. Neubauer's mission is to educate as many medical professionals as possible about the benefits of HBOT for children with cerebral palsy. In this way, he hopes to use his influence to hasten the time when HBOT becomes an accepted therapy for cerebral palsy.

INTRODUCTION

Parents and caregivers who are faced with the formidable prospect of caring for a child stricken with cerebral palsy or a brain injury often find themselves at a lack for resources when considering treatment options and determining the most effective course of action. This book was written with the purpose of bringing clarity to and providing accurate information concerning the use and value of hyperbaric oxygen therapy in the treatment of children who suffered oxygen deprivation before, during, or after birth. These include children who have experienced near-drowning, electrocution, traumatic brain injuries, cardiac arrest, carbon monoxide poisoning, and a multitude of other situations that can cause damage to the brain.

The term cerebral palsy (CP) refers to a spectrum of clinical neurological syndromes, characterized by abnormalities in movement and posture caused by a non-progressive insult to the immature brain. Both cerebral palsy and brain injury result from oxygen deprivation to the brain through inhibited blood circulation. Cerebral palsy is specifically defined as an early-onset disorder, occurring during the prenatal, perinatal, or immediate postnatal period. Causes of oxygen-deficiency are varied and not always apparent. Brain injuries are more broadly defined to include trauma (incurred through a variety of mediums, as stated above) occurring at any stage of life. The use of pressurized oxygen in the course of hyperbaric oxygen therapy, if administered in a timely fashion after the injury occurs, has been demonstrated to restore oxygenation to affected parts of the brain and to be instrumental in restoring brain function. This book is dedicated to the treatment and care of children with cerebral palsy or brain injuries, whose ages range from newly born to the mid-teens, or even perhaps beyond. It is of note that the oldest CP "child" who benefited from hyperbaric oxygen therapy was a 59-year-old Ph.D. in the United Kingdom. His main deficit was clarity of speech and after the treatments, for the first time in his life, he was able to communicate by telephone.

The book provides a comprehensive examination of the issues caregivers need to understand about hyperbaric oxygen therapy for children with cerebral palsy and brain injuries. While it is intended primarily for the caregivers of these children, the information will be of value to physicians, researchers, and insurance providers as well. This book covers a broad range of subjects from the functions of the brain to choosing a medically sound hyperbaric center where a child can receive appropriate treatments. One of the primary goals of the book is to demonstrate the positive effects of hyperbaric oxygen therapy (HBOT) so that each child's caregivers will understand and feel comfortable with the process and procedures of hyperbaric oxygen therapy. Another purpose is to help caregivers understand how activity in the brain is documented before and after HBOT through the use of single photon emission computed tomography (SPECT) scans.

Although there is now a great deal of data available on the internet on the subject of cerebral palsy and the use of HBO, and many caregivers are quite well informed on the subject (at times more so than their primary physicians), it often requires hours or even days to locate the exact, sought-after information. The object of this book is to incorporate most related information into one place. This information has been rendered in such a manner that it is both technically accurate and easy to understand. This book has been designed to guide caregivers through a logical series of chapters to facilitate their understanding of the role of hyperbaric oxygen therapy in helping children with cerebral palsy and brain injuries to function more effectively and develop more quickly. Each chapter discusses in depth a specific component of HBOT practices. While the book functions to provide a thorough and detailed account of every aspect of the therapy process from procuring treatment to followup care, its design also facilitates rapid access of information and allows the reader to use the book in the fashion that best suits his or her individual needs. Among the many other topics discussed, the book contains a section dedicated to answering the most common questions presented by caregivers, as well as a chapter providing an overview of hyperbaric oxygen therapy. As appropriate, information is cross-referenced, with a research section to provide assistance in gathering additional resources or in documenting any of the information included herein.

Case studies are presented throughout the book, including the testimonials of several parents and brief success stories about children who have received hyperbaric oxygen therapy. Additionally, the story of Rebecca, a five-year-old girl who has severe cerebral palsy is included in the center section of the book. This story, written by her dedicated father, will give all who have children with cerebral palsy or whose child has suffered a brain injury added hope and encouragement.

Extensive testing has demonstrated that in addition to physical, occupational, and speech therapies and appropriate medications, hyperbaric oxygen is one of the most effective therapies currently available for children with cerebral palsy or brain injuries. When properly administered over a period of time, hyperbaric oxygen therapy has been helpful to the majority of children treated. Of course, no type of therapy, no matter how effective, helps every child in the same way. Furthermore, sometimes a child may appear not to be noticeably improved when the therapy is first completed, but frequently, within a few weeks, the caregiver notices that progress is taking place. When children are helped to overcome their impairments, it enhances life. This type of small but significant change occurs on a daily basis in the lives of many children receiving hyperbaric oxygen therapy.

In the United States, the use of hyperbaric oxygen therapy for children with cerebral palsy and brain injuries is relatively new. This book provides an overview of the many years of work and discovery of this treatment modality. Hyperbaric oxygen therapy is an exciting and rapidly growing field. Every day, more is learned about the value of HBOT in the treatment of these children. Yet despite the many well-known specialists who are now prescribing HBOT as one of their chosen treatments for children with cerebral palsy and brain injuries, the lack of knowledge about the safety and value of HBOT by many U.S. physicians often deters parents from using it for their children. It is hoped that this book will help clarify the use of HBOT to caregivers as well as to the medical community.

Hyperbaric oxygen therapy is currently restricted to a set of very limited approved uses which will expand in time with further study and medical advances, but it is the ultimate hope of the author that all children afflicted with cerebral palsy or brain injuries will have access to the therapy they need to become as healthy, active, and productive as is within their means. This book will assist caregivers in obtaining the knowledge necessary to make sound judgments about the appropriateness of hyperbaric oxygen therapy in providing for the optimum health of the children in their care.

Richard A. Neubauer, M.D.
Medical Director, Ocean Hyperbaric Center
Lauderdale-by-the-Sea, Florida

OXYGEN: ITS IMPACT ON CEREBRAL PALSY AND BRAIN INJURIES

The positive power of the use of hyperbaric
oxygenation is really a modification of God's
gift to man—oxygen, the basis of life.
—Richard A. Neubauer, M.D.

Introduction

Understanding the role of oxygen in the human body is essential to a full comprehension of what frequently causes cerebral palsy and how hyperbaric oxygenation can play an important role in decreasing, or even ameliorating, the effects of cerebral palsy and brain injuries on the human body. Until one understands the effect of oxygen on the body, especially the brain, it can be difficult to see the relationship between hyperbaric oxygen therapy and cerebral palsy, or to discern how increasing the oxygen pressure in blood flowing to the brain can be of benefit in decreasing the symptoms of cerebral palsy.

First, it is essential to recognize that oxygen is the primary foundation for life. Man can survive for weeks without food, for days without water, but only minutes without oxygen. When oxygen is appropriately available to the critical parts of the body (the brain, heart, and lungs), it can mean the difference between life and death, coma and mental alertness, paralysis and movement, illness and health. When a portion of the brain is deprived of the correct amount of oxygen, any or all of the above conditions, as well as other impairments, may take place.

Second, the air the human body breathes is normally composed of 21 percent oxygen. Oxygen is carried throughout the body by red blood cells, which contain the binding factor hemoglobin. When oxygen is inhaled, the molecules dissolve in plasma and bind to the hemoglobin of red blood cells, which in turn carry oxygen to the body's tissues. Once oxygen has been transferred into the tissue, it is replaced with carbon dioxide (a waste product) that also binds to hemoglobin and is transported to the lungs where it is discharged. Thus, the delivery of oxygen under normal physiological circumstances requires appropriate circulation and is energy dependent at the cellular level.

Under conditions of hyperbaric oxygen, patients breathe 100% oxygen in a pressurized chamber. While pure oxygen is often referred to as a drug because it modulates some processes at different concentrations, oxygen under pressure is still the same gas that the body uses naturally. Under pressure there is increased penetration into tissues of the body. According to Henry's gas law of physics, oxygen under pressure will dissolve into body tissue and fluids in a direct proportion to the pressure used. Oxygen is thereby dissolved in the plasma, cells, bone, urine, blood, muscles, etc., and most importantly, cerebral spinal fluid.

This explains the significance of the statement by Edward Teller, Ph.D.,* that "hyperbaric oxygen delivers free molecular oxygen at the tissue level for immediate metabolic use without any energy exchange, even when the circulation is impaired."

In animal studies conducted by Dr. Ite Boerema, a Dutch physician, it was proven that hyperbaric oxygen can supply adequate amounts of oxygen to all organs of the body, even without blood. Under hyperbaric conditions, he replaced the blood circulating through pigs' bodies with saline solution. There was enough oxygen dissolved in other fluids of the body that the animals survived without any interruption of vital functions. Hemoglobin, carried by the red blood cells, is essential for the normal transport of oxygen, but from the standpoint of being the essential delivery system, it may be bypassed, at least on a temporary basis, if there is sufficient oxygen in the body fluids.

Oxygen: Man's Essential Element

Oxygen is a colorless, odorless gas that makes up about 21 percent of the atmosphere. All of the body's major components (water, protein, carbohydrates, fat) contain oxygen. The correct amount of oxygen in the body is essential to ensure that the body functions properly. When there is diminished oxygen in the body, all of the components function less efficiently.

* Dr. Teller developed the hydrogen bomb.

2

Under normal circumstances, the required oxygen flows through the body to the various parts (heart, lungs, stomach, brain, etc.) via the circulatory system. If there is any type of interruption of blood flow, it means that the amount of available oxygen, down to the capillaries and the tissues, may be seriously reduced. When the arterial flow is hindered, ischemia (loss of blood flow) and hypoxia (lack of oxygen) are the results.

Equally important, oxygen flowing through the blood brings about certain chemical reactions within the body that result in energy production. Energy is required for circulation, respiration, digestion, maintaining constant body temperature, and proper brain function. Only a minute amount of oxygen is required for normal intracellular chemical reactions to take place, and under normal circumstances, the rate of oxygen used is determined by the rate at which the respective cells expend energy. Energy production, aided by oxygen, is vitally important in the brain where the cells need adequate energy to generate the electrical activity that causes it to function properly.

Thus, oxygen is a critical element in the functioning of all parts of the body. If cells do not receive any oxygen, they die and may not be regenerated. On the other hand, if a cell is getting a small of amount of oxygen, it can remain viable for a much longer period than previously thought. In the case of the child with cerebral palsy or a traumatic brain injury, we are primarily interested in the brain cells (neurons), the length of time they remain viable, and how they can be revitalized.

Oxygen and the Brain

It is important to remember that the same facts regarding the need for oxygen to sustain life, and the time some cells may remain viable, are as true of neurons as any other cell in the body. The critical issue to remember when discussing cerebral palsy and other brain injuries is that if the mitichondria of certain cells do not receive enough oxygen to operate properly, but are receiving some oxygen, they may not die. In this case, hypoxia (underoxygenation of the tissues) occurs. It was scientifically proven in the mid-1980s that dormant brain cells can remain viable for many years. In the meantime, however, the diminished supply of oxygen causes multiple symptoms such as mental disturbances, shortness of breath, rapid pulse, fall in blood pressure, and, if there is a severe loss of oxygen, cyanosis (blueness of the skin and mucous membranes).

For the child diagnosed with cerebral palsy, when there is a loss of oxygen at or around the time of birth, there may eventually also be spasticity (stiffness), low muscle tone (hypotonia), and the loss of ability to move or control one or more muscle groups. Additionally, there may be related problems including speech disorders, impaired mental development, and seizures.

These same conditions are often in evidence when an older child or an adult receives a traumatic brain injury and incurs oxygen deprivation through choking, poisoning, near drowning, head injury, infections, reactions to immunization shots, or any other condition that causes brain damage. These brain injuries also result in a form of cerebral palsy not associated with birth. (Chapter 2)

Brief History of Hyperbaric Oxygen Therapy (HBOT)

The knowledge that hyperbaric oxygen treatment has a value to the body is not altogether new. Increased air pressure has been used for over a hundred years by the diving community to alleviate diving-related illnesses. The first actual use of air under pressure to treat decompression sickness was in 1848. Although those who used this pressurized air did not know it, the compressed air naturally boosted the oxygen content of the plasma.

The first practical hyperbaric chamber to investigate the therapeutic action of compression of air on maladies of the human body was designed, built, and described in writing by Junod in 1834. Junod was reported to have treated patients with a variety of medical problems, including paralysis, using compressed air. He is said to have gained highly beneficial results.

Other medical professionals and scientists who were instrumental in bringing about the present use and understanding of hyperbaric oxygen therapy are discussed later in this book. For our present discussion on oxygen, and oxygen at increased pressure, it is enough to understand that today it is common practice to use oxygen, administered in a hyperbaric chamber, for various illnesses and injuries. These include, but are certainly not limited to: air embolism, carbon monoxide intoxication, smoke inhalation, decompression illness, radiation myelitis, and treatment of wounds that will not heal. It is also becoming evident that other diseases such as multiple sclerosis (MS), Lyme disease, reflex sympathetic dystrophy (RSD), and many other disabling neurological conditions often show remarkable improvement following hyperbaric oxygen therapy treatments.

A Tragic Medical Mistake

Since the early 1950s, when surface oxygen was mistakenly thought to cause retrolental fibroplasia (blindness) in premature babies, the incidence of cerebral palsy has risen dramatically in the United States. The reason for not giving oxygen (normobaric) to the hypoxic (low oxygen) neonate or premature baby is that surface oxygen was thought to cause this type of blindness. Consequently, a medical procedure was established that limited the amount of oxygen a newborn could receive to 40%.

Clinical studies have since proven that it was not the use of increased oxygen that caused the vision problems. Rather, it was the early withdrawal of the infant from the oxygen environment that caused the problem. As early as 1951, Szewezyk suggested that retrolental fibroplasia resulted from initially habituating a child to an enriched oxygen environment and then suddenly withdrawing the child from it. By 1964, Forrester also reported that retinopathy developed upon withdrawal from the high level of oxygen. He found that the best thing to do was to reintroduce the child to the oxygen environment. His report stated that a slow reduction of oxygen and final return to the atmospheric concentration for several weeks was all that was necessary to cure the problem. In some instances, repeated sessions with increased oxygen have actually resolved the situation.

This was confirmed through research by Dr. P.B. James of Dundee, Scotland, in the 1990s. He brought to light serious misinterpretations of multicenter studies regarding surface oxygen and retrolental fibroplasia.

Although this fallacy has existed for nearly 50 years, and is still being perpetuated in many medical schools, the use of hyperbaric oxygen does not produce this effect. It is unfortunate that many children in the United States who are hypoxic at birth are not given the opportunity for increased oxygen therapy to correct their condition. It is now standard practice, however, in many countries including Russia, China, Cuba, South America, and parts of Mexico to give hypoxic children increased oxygen under pressure. Additionally, there is a major teaching center in New York that is, on occasion, taking the hypoxic or potentially brain-injured baby (3 - 12 hours old) to the hyperbaric chamber. Current international studies are demonstrating that the incidence of cerebral palsy is dramatically less in those situations where it is standard procedure to give hypoxic infants increased oxygen.

The Role of HBOT

To the majority of the medical profession, hyperbaric oxygen therapy is a relatively new therapy to help children with cerebral palsy or a brain injury overcome the debilitating conditions that are consistent with neurological damage. Yet this treatment is both well recognized and consistent with healing and aiding other wounds.

Hyperbaric oxygen is the delivery of 100% pure oxygen at greater than atmospheric pressure through the use of a hyperbaric chamber. [This is referred to as ATA (absolute atmospheres) in discussing hyperbaric oxygen therapy.] The pressure can be administered in ranges from 1.1 to 3 ATA using 100 percent oxygen or up to 6 ATA using compressed air. This last type of treatment is listed in certain U.S. Navy diving tables.

Even lower pressures may be needed if seizure activity is present. Under these circumstances, pressures of 1.1 to 1.25 ATA using 100 percent oxygen are appropriate. This frequently effectively treats the seizure disorder and thereby helps to reduce or stop ancillary medications.

The Effects of HBOT on the Brain

It has long been understood that healing cannot be achieved without sufficient levels of oxygen in the tissues where illness and injuries take place and often linger. Traditionally, injuries to the brain often have been the hardest "wounds" to heal. Until the discovery that hyperbaric oxygen therapy would assist brain injuries in the same way it helps other tissue injuries, there was little that could be done to "repair" or "jump start" the brain. There were merely various types of therapy and medications to help reduce the effects of trauma after the injury or illness was over.

K.K. Jain in *The Textbook of Hyperbaric Medicine* states, "The most important metabolic effects of hyperbaric oxygenation are on the brain." One of the most important studies on the pressure to be used for treatment of cerebral disorders is the study conducted by Holbach, et al. in 1977. This study found that the optimal pressure for treating patients with brain injuries is 1.5 ATA because the cerebral glucose metabolism is balanced at this pressure.

Generally, hyperbaric oxygen therapy is safe and well tolerated by humans at 1.5 - 2 ATA. In Canada, certain medical centers, operating as hyperbaric centers, routinely use 1.75 ATA at 100 percent oxygen for children with cerebral palsy and brain injuries. For this reason, a few medically operated hyperbaric centers in the United States give 1.75 oxygen tension to children with cerebral palsy and brain injuries as well. The Holbach study further noted that "No adverse effects are seen at 1.5 ATA for exposures up to 40 - 60 minutes."

Another important study conducted in 1999 by a group of medical professionals at McGill University in Quebec, Canada has indicated that while hyperbaric oxygen therapy is effective for children with cerebral palsy, 1.5 ATA pressurized oxygen may not be needed. The control group treated with 1.3 ATA pressurized air appeared to have received similar benefits as the 1.75 pressurized oxygen ATA group, although the 1.75 ATA group had better and faster results. In this study, the results of the 40 treatments of therapy were still in effect for all participants, and even after three months experienced no regression. Further studies are underway including one at Cornell University.

Oxygen Toxicity

Like all treatments involving a drug, even a natural one, it is possible to give or take too much. In treatment with oxygen this is known as oxygen toxicity, which can occur when oxygen is administered in large doses, causing seizures, irreversible neurological damage, or even death. It has been established through many scientific research experiments that 3-hour exposures at 3 ATA or a 30 - 40 minute exposure at 4 ATA is where the danger point begins. For this reason, hyperbaric oxygen therapy in children never goes beyond 2 ATA for neurologic conditions, the point at which pure oxygen ceases to be of benefit. Higher pressures such as 6 ATA are used exclusively for the treatment of divers. At this ATA, pressurized air, not pure oxygen, is used.

It is agreed that the optimum pressure for the treatment of chronic brain injuries in children is between 1.3 ATA and 1.75 ATA using pure oxygen. It is postulated that oxygen toxicity may be further prevented by administering supplemental vitamins E and C prior to treatment. If oxygen toxicity does indeed occur, it can frequently be simply brought under control by a reduction in pressure or by changing the breathing gas from oxygen to air.

In comparison to clinical and animal data on the use of hyperbaric oxygen therapy for many types of injury and illness, there is relatively little data published in the United States on the effects of hyperbaric oxygen therapy for children with cerebral palsy or other traumatic brain insults. Nevertheless, a number of centers in other countries are using hyperbaric oxygen therapy with dramatic results for thousands of children with cerebral palsy.

How Increased Oxygen Helps

It has been suggested that hyperbaric oxygen therapy may have positive effects on "idling neurons" that have been disabled by the initial insult and are not working to their full capacity. The use of hyperbaric oxygen therapy has been shown to activate these cells. This will be discussed in detail later in this book.

Consider these two cases:

Jason was diagnosed with cerebral palsy shortly after birth. At seven years of age, he had a vocabulary of only ten words and the mental level of a two- to three-year-old. He had never learned to walk and still crawled. After 61 hyperbaric treatments, he could walk with assistance, and had improved in every way, both cognitively and in his motor skills. Nothing had changed in his life except the addition of hyperbaric treatments.

Rebecca was pronounced "brain-dead" for 35 minutes after her birth, but survived after being taken off life support. She is a severe cerebral palsy patient, but is mentally very alert. One of her physical problems was the inability to swallow anything that was thin liquid. All of her beverages had to be thickened with commercial thickeners. After only six hyperbaric treatments, Rebecca could swallow thin liquids, including water.

Of course, not all patients enjoy such dramatic benefits from hyperbaric therapy, but most caregivers welcome the opportunity to give their loved ones every chance for improvement. While hyperbaric oxygen therapy is NOT a miracle cure, it does offer new hope for many neurologically damaged children, because the results achieved are proving to be effective, safe, non-invasive, and permanent.

Here's an important question to consider:
Q. What can I (the reader) do to help?

A. Become informed about the value of hyperbaric oxygen therapy, join a parents' advocacy group, and make certain your primary doctor and specialists become totally informed about the scientific data on the subject. (Chapter 10)

HBOT and Insurance Companies

The United States is lagging behind many other countries in their research of the use of hyperbaric therapy. This brings us to a commonly asked question:

Q. When will most major insurance companies begin to pay for hyperbaric oxygen therapy?

A. When there is documented evidence (through controlled, double-blind studies) that proves its medical value or by governmental legislation. (Chapter 10)

This lack of controlled, double-blind studies is critical for children with cerebral palsy and other traumatic brain insults. (Double-Blind studies consist of experiments or clinical trials in which neither the subjects nor the researchers know which subjects are receiving the active treatment and which are not.) It is also questionably ethical to perform double-blind studies in children. It should also be noted that there is no medical standard of care for CP and the brain-injured child, therefore even commonly prescribed modalities of therapy and many drugs must be considered experimental. Until the United States medical profession accepts the value of hyperbaric oxygen therapy for these children, many of the primary doctors will not prescribe it or support it. Many medical professionals will continue to tell caregivers that such treatment won't help the child. This makes it easy for insurance companies to deny payment for therapy, and puts the responsibility of paying for treatment solely on the shoulders of the individual caregivers.

Conclusion

There is scientific evidence that some cells in the brain, specifically neurons which have been damaged by various insults, may be dormant, but alive for as long as 14 years after the incident. There is additional scientific evidence (through the use of SPECT scans, see Chapter 6) that increasing oxygen delivery in a hyperbaric chamber can "awaken" dormant cells in some cerebral palsy and brain injured children. There is an increasing amount of evidence through clinical studies, semi-blind studies, and observations that many cerebral palsy and brain injured children, worldwide, have improved mentally, physically, and emotionally after a dose (40+ treatments) or more of hyperbaric oxygen treatments.

CEREBRAL PALSY / TRAUMATIC BRAIN INJURIES: ENEMIES OF CHILDREN

Often in life we are provided with the opportunity to positively influence others while helping ourselves. I believe that hyperbaric oxygen therapy is the key to a brighter future and improved quality of life for many brain injured children. I share this belief with parents everywhere.

—Claudine Lanoix (Nadeau)
mother of five, including
twins with CP

Introduction

While it is often difficult to determine the causes of brain damage, it has now been proven in clinical studies that a primary problem is the lack of proper oxygenation of brain cells. Sometimes these cells (neurons) that are not functioning are not dead, but merely idling or dormant. When hyperbaric oxygen therapy (HBOT) is properly administered, it often helps to stimulate these living but nonfunctional brain cells.

Cerebral Palsy Defined

Cerebral palsy is a "catch-all" term that encompasses many etiological factors in children up to age 14. "Cerebral" refers to the brain and "palsy" to muscle weakness / poor control. As the name implies, in most instances, the term cerebral palsy describes a varied group of chronic conditions that affect the movement of the body and the coordination of muscles. The problems associated with cerebral palsy and other neurodevelopmental disorders may present *in utero*, perinatal, or postnatal. The condition has a wide variety of characteristics that may be present at birth or may not become apparent for months...or until the occurrence of a head injury or some other medical cause.

Most frequently, cerebral palsy is diagnosed between the ages of 6 and 12 months when it becomes apparent that the child is not making appropriate strides in physical development. It is not progressive (i.e., does not get worse), although secondary conditions sometimes develop which may improve, worsen, or remain the same over time. It is not communicable, and in the truest sense, it is not a disease. It is damage to the child's brain that results in difficulties in motor control, and often interferes with learning and living normally. Currently, the disorder affects about 2 of every 1,000 live births. It occurs in all socioeconomic groups, races, and countries. In about 70% - 80% of the cases, the reasons for the defects in the brain cannot be determined with absolute certainty, but one of the primary causes is known to be prolonged oxygen deprivation.

Causes of Cerebral Palsy

As previously noted, the causes of cerebral palsy are multiple, including uterine problems, complications at time of delivery, post-delivery infections, trauma, genetic predisposition, vaccinations, congenital abnormalities, aneurysms, intra-cerebral hemorrhage, and mulitfactorial etiology. It is also known to have been caused by hypoxia, ischemia, infection, metabolic derangement and deficiencies, or serious illnesses with high fevers. The common denominator in nearly all cases of cerebral palsy is some degree of brain damage because of an insufficient amount of oxygen reaching the fetal, newborn, or young brain.

There are a number of reasons why the oxygen supply to the brain may be interrupted. A few of the most frequent causes are: premature separation of the placenta from the walls of the uterus, low birth weight, Rh or A-B-O blood incompatibility between mother and child, position of the baby during birth, change of pressure if the baby is born too quickly or too slowly, interference with circulation in the umbilical cord, infections to the mother during pregnancy, premature birth with immature pulmonary systems, and microorganisms that attack the infant's nervous system.

A partial list of causes and the times of their occurrence include the following:

Prenatal Causes	**(In the womb)**
Anoxia	Problems with the umbilical cord
Intrauterine Infections	
Metabolic Disorders	Diabetes, heart condition, hyperthyroidism, asthma
Rh Factor	Rh sensitization
Abdominal Injury	Car accident, falls, traumas
Prenatal care	Insufficient or absent prenatal care
Virus Infections	German measles (rubella), toxoplasmosis, herpes simplex

Perinatal Causes	**(During and immediately after delivery)**
Anoxia	Umbilical cord distress or misplacement
Asphyxia	Mechanical respiratory obstruction
Analgesis	Drugs that affect the respiratory system
Delivery Problems	Breech, hemorrhaging
Pressure changes	Delivery too abrupt or too slow
Premature	Low birth weight, underdeveloped lungs
Trauma	Use of forceps

Acquired Cerebral Palsy	**(Ages 1 - 3)**
Anoxia	Strangulation, carbon monoxide poisoning, near-drowning, near-hanging, smoke inhalation
Infections	High fevers, meningitis, encephalitis, brain abscess
Neoplasms	Cysts, tumors, hydrocephalus
Vascular Problems	Hemorrhage, thrombosis
Trauma	Falls, head injuries, gun shots, fractures, accidents, shaken baby syndrome

Conditions Related to Cerebral Palsy

Whatever the initial cause, and depending on what part of the brain has been affected, a number of impairments can occur. Some of the more common symptoms parents notice as the child grows older are muscle spasm or tightness, involuntary movements, and dysfunction in mobility and gait. Other conditions that occur with a great deal of regularity include seizures or epilepsy (ongoing, regular, frequent seizures of any degree); mental retardation; impairment of hearing, sight, and speech; abnormal sensation and perception; problems related to feeding, bladder, and bowel control; and mild to severe learning disabilities.

All children with cerebral palsy have problems with muscle tone, either with the stretch and resistance or the give and take of their muscles. Some children have muscles that are floppy and relaxed (hypotonic), and other children have muscles that are abnormally tight (hypertonic). Some children have fluctuating muscle tone, which creates involuntary movements, tremors, or variation in the strength and weakness of the muscles during an intentional movement. Each of these types of muscle tone can have dramatic effects on the development of fine and gross motor skills.

Diagnosis of Cerebral Palsy

The diagnosis of cerebral palsy (CP) is often made by the child's pediatrician based on the child's inability to fully control muscle movements. Symptoms and signs that parents can look for include: early sucking difficulty with breast or bottle, lack of normal muscle tone (early), slow development (walking and talking), unusual body postures, stiffness (later), stiffness and muscle spasms, purposeless body movements, poor coordination or balance, crossed eyes, deafness, convulsions, and various degrees of mental retardation (as the child grows older).

Classifications of Cerebral Palsy

The problems of each child are unique, but there are several general classifications (types) of cerebral palsy, each reflecting the distribution of the injury and the nature of the motor impairment. The three primary classifications are:

Pyramidal (Spastic) – Spastic cerebral palsy is the most common type. It affects more than 75% of all children with cerebral palsy. Children have one or more tight muscle groups which cause them to make stiff and difficult movements. The symptoms of this type of cerebral palsy include exaggerated stretch reflexes, contractions or abnormal shortenings of muscles and tendons around joints, ankle clonus, persistent primary reflexes, and positive Babinski (a reflex extension of the great toe with flexion of the other toes, evoked by stroking the sole of the foot—normal in infants but otherwise denoting damage to the central nervous system).

If a child has spastic cerebral palsy, it is because there has been damage to the motor cortex—the part of the brain that controls voluntary movements—or to the white matter through which the motor output from the cortex travels before arriving at the spine and muscles.

Extrapyramidal (Choreo-athetoid) – This category of cerebral palsy affects approximately 5 - 15% of children with cerebral palsy. When this part of the child's brain is impacted, the child usually exhibits involuntary movements that have no purpose. Because the areas most affected are the face, arms, and trunk, the child often has difficulty with speaking, feeding, reaching, or grasping. The lack of muscle tone in the trunk makes it difficult for the child to maintain the posture needed for sitting up, crawling, or walking. The most common terms given to these symptoms are:

Dystonia	slow, twising, rhythmic movements
Athetosis	slow, writhing movements
Chorea	abrupt, jerky movements in the head area
Ataxia	lack of coordination in standing and walking
Rigidity	extremely high muscle tone
Dyskinesia	generalized involuntary movements

This type of cerebral palsy is caused by damage to the cerebellum or basal ganglia. These are the areas of the brain which process the signals for smooth, coordinated movements and correct posture. These involuntary and uncontrolled movements are often not apparent until the child is between six and nine months old when normal development would usually include rolling over, sitting up, etc.

Mixed-Type Cerebral Palsy – This is the type of cerebral palsy wherein a child experiences the spastic movements and the involuntary movements of both pyramidal and extrapyramidal cerebral palsy.

Another common term used with children with cerebral palsy is ataxia—a disturbed sense of balance and depth perception. Furthermore, depending on which part of the child's body is affected by the problems associated with movement, they will be further classified as follows:

Monoplegia	only one limb on one side of the body (very rare)
Diplegia	affects mainly the child's legs
Hemiplegia	affects only one side of the body; usually the arm is the most affected

Quadriplegia affects the child's whole body; legs can be more affected than arms. Because of the extent of the motor disability, most of life's activities are affected

Another term that is frequently used has the same meaning as quadriplegia:

Double Hemiplegia affects the child's whole body; arms most affected,with major feeding and speech impairments

Any of these types can vary from slightly clumsy to total paralysis. There seems to be no specific degree of motor problems associated with any specific type.

Hemiplegia—the involvement of one side of the body—indicates damage to the opposite cerebral hemisphere. In diplegic cerebral palsy, the type most often seen with children born prematurely, the arms are usually less affected than the legs. The most severe form of cerebral palsy is quadriplegia. This type of CP involves mass cerebral damage to multiple parts of the brain and most parts of the body are affected to some degree.

Therapy Modalities

At this time, the primary treatment modalities for children with cerebral palsy are physical therapy, occupational therapy, and different aspects of speech therapy. Starting as soon as possible after the child has been diagnosed with a developmental disorder, most modalities try to help the child and the caregiver "manage" the disorder. Therapies may involve helping the child learn to deal with vision and hearing problems as well as social and emotional development. Physicians, therapists, nurses, social workers, caregivers, and often educators are involved in this management process.

All in all, these modalities are geared at helping the child achieve maximum potential in growth and development, but do not intend to change the physical brain function of the child. This is where the use of hyperbaric oxygen therapy (HBOT) differs completely. The goal of HBOT is to reactivate cells in the child's brain that are alive but non-functional, and to assist the child in recovery from some of the damage brought on by lack of sufficient oxygen to the brain. At the same time, the child continues all of the other therapies previously mentioned, as it has been determined through clinical studies that active learning is needed to keep new brain cells excited and working.

> DW was a three-year-old male who suffered perinatal hypoxic ischemic encephalopathy with renal failure consisting of acute tubular necrosis, thromocytopenia, sepsis, respiratory insufficiency, hypo-volemia, and apnea related to a seizure order. It is remarkable that he survived with all of these medical problems. After receiving 21 treatments of hyperbaric oxygen therapy, he was able to sit up and hold a cup for the first time in his life. He was more attentive, made new vocal sounds, was more aware of his surroundings, and began to grab at everything. With these new capabilities, he was a prime candidate for physical, occupational, and speech therapy.

The standard, recognized therapies for children with cerebral palsy such as physical, occupational, and speech therapies are usually insurance-covered services. For the most part, these therapies focus on improving mobility. Other interventions that also focus on mobility include medications and, in a limited number of cases, surgeries. While most children are assisted by these therapeutic interventions to some degree, progress is often quite slow. Unfortunately, the other disabilities a child may have most often have the greatest impact on what the child can and can't do. As yet, the standard, recognized therapies have not shown much success in working with learning disabilities, vision problems, or complex motor conditions such as swallowing.

Additionally, it is interesting to note that these therapies are not based on any clinical research including controlled, blind studies. The rationale for the lack of scientific, clinical studies of the therapies listed above is that it is quite difficult to establish a control and a non-control group because every child's case is unique. Furthermore, it is offensive to ask parents to spend time and energy with their children in a study where at least one-half of the children are not going to benefit by the experience. The same is true of the medication used to decrease spasticity or seizures. No one wants to give a child a placebo when he or she needs medication to reduce both of these conditions.

Long-term Effects of Cerebral Palsy

Dr. Maurine Packard of Cornell University conducted a small, randomized, delayed-entry trial of the effects of hyperbaric oxygen therapy on children aged 1 to 5 with cerebral palsy. She reported that the problems with cerebral palsy often extend far beyond motor control. In the findings of her study, she recognized a report compiled by Kuban and Leviton in 1994. This study found that nearly half of children with cerebral palsy are reported as mentally retarded, one-fourth have learning disabilities, and about one-third have seizures. Many of the involvements are severe enough to interfere with activities of daily living.

The long-term prognosis for those with cerebral palsy is quite poor. A United States government study on the independent living status of individuals with cerebral palsy found that only 30%—the least affected adults—are able to live alone as financially independent individuals. For the most part, these individuals have normal intelligence, are ambulatory, and do not have seizures. According to a NINDS (National Institute of Neurological Disorders and Strokes) publication, the estimated cost of taking care of individuals with cerebral palsy in the United States is five billion dollars annually. It is this type of cost and the discouraging future predicted for most children with cerebral palsy that we hope to change through the use of hyperbaric oxygen therapy.

Responses of Cerebral Palsy Associations to HBOT

Interestingly, it is the lack of controlled studies that many physicians, insurance companies, and the leading cerebral palsy associations give as their primary reason for not recommending hyperbaric oxygen therapy (HBOT). They say they are waiting for controlled, double-blinded clinical trials to prove the effectiveness of increased oxygen tension. There is also concern that reports on the use of HBOT are primarily anecdotal. That is, the observations of caregivers, the child's therapists, and, perhaps, the child's primary doctor about the progress the child has made serve as the rationale for determining the success of HBOT for the individual child. While such observation is not as scientific as a controlled, blinded study would be, it is the method most often used to determine the success of other therapy modalities.

The most positive statement yet published from the American Academy for Cerebral Palsy and Developmental Medicine, the United Cerebral Palsy Research and Educational Foundation, and the United Cerebral Palsy

Associations came in their September 1999 report on the *Present Status of Hyperbaric Oxygen Therapy for the Treatment of Cerebral Palsy:* "Although not yet demonstrated, it is conceivable that hyperbaric oxygenation may be of help to selected persons with certain kinds of disabilities." They write in the same article that "There is no scientifically acceptable evidence available at this time that demonstrates its [HBOT's] clinical usefulness; neither is there any scientifically acceptable evidence available at this time demonstrating its lack of usefulness."

While this is certainly not the clinical evidence these groups say must be presented, it should be noted that they are adopting a "wait and see" attitude. In the meantime, there is clear evidence of the improvement of many children with cerebral palsy after they receive a series of HBO treatments. This documentation has been made using each patient as "his or her own control."

Support of NINDS

Much of the research conducted on neurological diseases and traumas conducted in the United States since the 1950s has been made possible through the support of the National Institute of Neurological Disorders and Strokes (NINDS), the leading supporter of neurological research in the United States. The controlled studies to document findings have been carried out in both private and public institutions. Overall, NINDS has supported research on more than 600 neurological diseases (muscular dystrophy), developmental disorders (cerebral palsy), degenerative diseases of adults (Alzheimer's disease), metabolic diseases (Gaucher's disease), cerebrovascular diseases (stroke), convulsive diseases (epilepsy), infectious diseases (AIDS dementia), brain tumors, and trauma (spinal cord and head injuries).

Research conducted by NINDS ranges from studies on the structure and function of single brain cells to tests of new diagnostic tools and treatments for those with neurological disorders. It is hoped that in the very near future this group may find the funding necessary to clearly demonstrate the value of hyperbaric oxygen therapy for children with cerebral palsy and brain injuries. This would be of tremendous benefit to many children who are not yet able to be treated with this safe, non-invasive form of therapy. It would complement and confirm many of the studies that are being carried out in other countries, including the UK, Canada, China, Russia, Slovenia, Bulgaria, Cuba, and South America.

Studies in these countries are clinically proving the effectiveness of hyperbaric oxygen therapy for cerebral palsy and traumatic brain insults.

The Value of HBOT for Children with Brain Injuries

Even without definitive scientific evidence, many caregivers have found HBOT to be highly effective. In many cases, it is not just "word-of-mouth" evidence that supports the changes in children. In many centers, videos have been used to document changes in children before and after hyperbaric treatments. In these videos, patients are assessed for visual and cognitive abilities, fine and gross motor changes, and positive changes in spasticity. One of the most thrilling responses for parents is the increased awareness and attention that became apparent in treated children. This is a behavior that is difficult to measure, but easy for the caregiver to notice. This may be considered anecdotal, but at this time, it is the best proof available. This is not to say that clinical studies are not needed; they are. This is especially true in the United States where support of the entire medical and insurance industries is sorely needed and depends on the results of clinical studies.

Worldwide Research

Chapter 10 provides a short overview of some of the most recent studies being conducted worldwide. When the findings of these scientific studies are combined with the videos and observations of physicians and caregivers, it makes a very strong statement about the value of HBOT for children with cerebral palsy and traumatic brain injuries.

Since the 1970s, HBOT has been used worldwide to treat thousands of patients with chronic brain injuries. SPECT (single photon emission computed tomography) scans have clearly proven that "hyperbaric oxygen not only relieves hypoxia, but also 'jump-starts' the brain to much better organization and function." Through the use of SPECT scans, it is possible to determine which part of the brain is not functioning properly and has decreased metabolism. The SPECT scan can be used before and after hyperbaric oxygen therapy treatments to discover positive changes in functions in the parts of the brain where activity was diminished.

Current studies from other countries are increasingly offering evidence that in the very young, hyperbaric oxygen therapy produces a better milieu for the growth of new brain tissue. For many years, physicians in Russia, China, Japan, Italy, and some South American countries have been taking hypoxic or neurologically impaired infants from the delivery room to the hyperbaric chamber. Their studies report clinical effects that are remarkable. It has also been shown to assist children when given at a later time. There is more and more evidence that hyperbaric oxygenation not only relieves hypoxia, but also "jumpstarts" the brain to much better organization and function.

> JS, a full-term boy whose delivery was complicated by prolonged cord constriction of the neck, seizures, subdural hematoma, and traumatic intubation, developed cerebral palsy. The initial SPECT scan at 15 months showed multiple marked areas of hypoperfusion. He received 35 HBOTs at 1.5 ATA, 1 - 2 per day, 5 - 6 days per week, over a time period of 22 days. Repeat SPECT scan after 35 HBOT treatments showed considerable improvement. The patient experienced better gross motor and head control, standing balance, decreased spacticity, was drinking out of a cup, and had increased vocalization.

Cost of HBOT

There is also the question of the cost of the hyperbaric oxygen therapy. Currently, the majority of expenses are being paid personally by the caregivers and their friends and families. A quick comparison of the cost of "lifetime" care versus HBO treatments indicates that the care of a brain injured child, including medication, hospitalization, special trans-portation vehicles, paid caregivers, education, therapies, and changes to the home usually is in the millions of dollars over the lifetime of the individual. In contrast, a complete series of hyperbaric treatments would cost a maximum of $300,000. More importantly, there is the chance that the child could recover much of the use of his or her brain rather than just having managed care.

Regardless of whether society or the family is paying the bills, the difference in costs is remarkable. It would seem that society, as well as caregivers, should have an interest in finding out if HBOT is effective …if only from a financial outlook. Perhaps this should be brought to the attention of legislators who can help resolve such discrepancies in payment allowed for children with special needs. If HBOT is helping a child with cerebral palsy or a brain injury, why is this cost not covered as are other types of therapy? In fact, few, if any, of the therapies for children with cerebral palsy have been scientifically proven through double-blind studies. Furthermore, only 17% of Medicare insurance reimbursement conditions have been documented with this type of study.

Conclusion

Thus, while the causes of cerebral injury can result from conditions that the mother incurs before or during pregnancy, traumas during or shortly after the delivery, premature birth, or childhood injuries, the common thread is damage to the brain, often caused by hypoxia (lack of oxygen) to the brain cells. It is hoped that scientific data from around the world, as well as the United States, will clearly demonstrate that children with hypoxia should be treated immediately (even in the womb) rather than wait for devastating changes to occur in the brain. It is always more medically sound to use preventative measures rather than try to repair damages.

For children with cerebral palsy, hyperbaric oxygen therapy is a very viable option. For many children, there have been noteworthy dramatic improvements in functional brain imaging paralleling clinical improvement. While certainly not a cure-all, HBOT has the potential of helping the child acquire the use of brain cells that have been living, but lacking the "electrical spark" needed to make them function properly.

When starved for oxygen and nutrients, nerve cells in the brain selectively shut down electrical functions to save energy. This reserves the energy available for more critical cellular functions such as pumping out toxins and keeping an electrolytic balance within the cell membrane. If these idle, lethargic cells are restored to appropriate oxygen levels, they may return to normalcy and once again become electrically active. When this happens, there is a corresponding positive reaction in bodily functions. Sometimes the cells need "retraining" in order to become totally functional. For this reason, it is recommended that the child continue with physical, speech, and occupational therapy modalities to ensure that the newly awakened brain cells "learn" new skills and activities.

One of the primary responsibilities of the caregiver who is considering HBOT treatments for the child is to be certain that the center administering the therapy is medically sound and properly operated. (Chapter 8)

22

THE MAGNIFICENT BRAIN

*The magnificent human brain is the creator of all of
man's thoughts, emotions, words, and deeds.*

—J. Scott Lee

Introduction

Learning new things about the brain and how it functions is an on-going challenge to scientists and the medical profession, but it is not a new venture. Man has been making discoveries for more than three centuries, and recent years have seen a period of rapid progress. The decade of the 1990s was declared the *Decade of the Brain* by the United States Congress because scientists learned more about the brain in those 10 years than had been learned in all the previous centuries of study. This progress was made possible by the increasing pace of new research techniques, technology, and the growth in neurological and behavioral sciences. New information gives children with cerebral palsy and brain injuries a greater chance to overcome some of the difficulties to which they have been forced to adapt.

David suffered a stroke due to a traumatic birth, which left him with a large infarction [a localized area of tissue that is dying or dead, having been deprived of its blood supply] in the left hemisphere of his brain. At age 3 1/2, he functioned at about a 10 - 15 month level. He had cognitive and motor disabilities, and spent most of his time in a wheelchair. After 193 HBOT treatments, David showed dramatic improvements in all areas of his life and was able "to run all over the place." His brain function is now much improved due to hyperbaric oxygen therapy.

Importance of the Brain

The brain is the center of intelligence. It interprets the senses, it is the initiator of body movement, and it controls behavior. It is by far the most complex part of the human body, and the one area that can cause the most impact on normal functions when it is not operating properly. It is the source of all the activities that define what a person can and cannot do.

When the brain is healthy, it functions quickly and automatically, and most people give little thought to how it operates or which part of the brain is responsible for each of the many functions it controls. When brain damage or traumatic injury occurs, however, the results of the brain not operating properly can be devastating to the individual involved. Knowing more about the brain and how it operates is an effective way to help understand how and why such problems occur when there is a brain injury.

This basic understanding of the brain, and how injuries affect its normal processing, also makes it easier to understand the role hyperbaric oxygen therapy plays in correcting the problem. It will also facilitate an appreciation of the role of increased oxygen tension on the cells of the brain.

The brain is such a complex organ that it would be impossible in one short chapter to explain all that it does and how it operates. Therefore, the explanation given here is a rather simple one. Its purpose is to briefly explain how the brain functions when it is healthy and what happens when the brain is diseased or dysfunctional.

Composition of the Brain

Each part of the brain has its own special properties and responsibilities, but each part is often dependent on the actions of other parts to operate at its optimum. Composed of three parts, one section of the brain often co-mingles with another part or parts to effectively deliver the services it provides to various parts of the body. When there is a brain injury, regardless of what part of the brain is affected, there may be residual damage or infarction to other parts of the brain as well.

The three separate parts of the brain are located within the skull as indicated by the shaded areas in the diagram below:

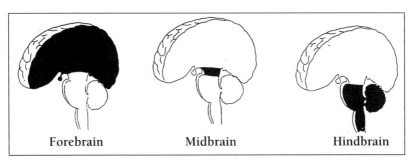

Forebrain   Midbrain   Hindbrain

FIGURE A-1

The Forebrain	The Midbrain	The Hindbrain
The largest and most developed part of the brain	Controls reflex actions	Upper part of spinal cord Brain stem Cerebellum
Primarily contains the cerebrum	Partially controls voluntary movements	Operates learned rote movements (such as hitting a baseball or playing the trumpet)
Encloses the inner brain		Controls vital functions, including respiration and heart beat

Figure A-2 depicts the different parts of the brain. There are nine major areas of the brain which are on the exterior. (Other parts of the brain are hidden inside an area called the inner brain, as illustrated in Figure A-3.)

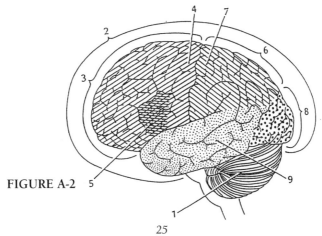

FIGURE A-2

The chart below is a simplified explanation of the role of each area of the brain. (Each part has additional responsibilities that integrate the various activities of one section of the brain with another section.)

The outer brain consists of:

Name	Function(s)
1. Cerebellum	Rote movements.
2. Cerebrum	Intellectual activities: holds memories, allows imagination, thinking, recognizing friends, reading, playing games. There are two hemispheres split by a deep fissure; they communicate with each other through a thick tract of nerve fibers at their base. They are a mirror image of each other, but have very different functions. Left hemisphere: ability to form words. Right hemisphere: abstract reasoning skills.
3. Frontal lobes (2)	Planning, imagining the future, reasoned arguments (short term storage area).
4. Motor area (rear of frontal lobes)	Helps control voluntary movement.
5. Broca's area (left frontal lobe)	Allows thoughts to be transformed into words.
6. Parietal lobes (posterior area)	Taste, aroma, and texture of foods.
7. Parietal lobes (anterior area)	Sensory areas; taste, touch, temperature, movement; information from the rest of the body. Also reading and arithmetic.
8. Occipital lobes	Processes images from the eyes; links information with images stored in the memory. Damage causes blindness.
9. Temporal lobes (in front of viscial area)	Receives information from the ears; forms and receives memories, especially associated with music.

The Inner Brain

The inner brain is composed of the hypothalamus, thalamus, hippocampus, and ganglia.

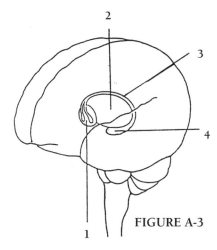

FIGURE A-3

The inner brain is located deep within the interior of the brain, and its three parts serve as the "gatekeepers" between the spinal cord and the cerebral hemispheres. These structures determine the emotional status of an individual and modify responses and perceptions. They also allow people to initiate movements without actually thinking about each movement (such as driving the car or brushing your teeth).

Name	Function
1. Hypothalamus	About the size of a pearl, it wakes you in the morning, makes the adrenaline flow (fight or flight), and controls molecules for anger, sadness, or exhilaration.
2. Thalamus	Major communication center for information going to and from the spinal cord and the cerebrum. Surrounding the thalamus is a cluster of nerves called the basal ganglia which are responsible for initiating and integrating movement. When the nerve cells that lead into the basal ganglia are diseased it causes tremors, rigidity, and a stiff, shuffling walk (i.e., Parkinson's disease).
3. Ganglia	Leads from the hypothalamus and/or to the hippocampus.
4. Hippocampus	The memory index; sends memories to appropriate parts of the cerebral hemisphere for long-term storage. Retrieves memories as needed.

The cerebrum and the cerebellum are coated with a layer of tissue about one-eighth-inch thick, sometimes slightly less. This vital layer of tissue called the cortex (Latin for bark) is where most of the actual information processing takes place. The term "gray matter" refers to this part of the brain because it does not have the same protective insulation that gives the rest of the brain a white color. More information can be processed than would seem possible at first glance because the folds in this part of the brain add to the surface area and increase the "gray matter."

For reasons as yet unknown to scientists, most of the signals from the brain to the body, and from the body to the brain, cross over on their way to and from the brain. Thus, the right cerebral hemisphere controls the left side of the body and vice versa. When one side of the brain is damaged, the opposite side of the body is usually most affected.

All parts of the brain are composed of a number of different types of cells. The most important cell, and the only one discussed in this book, is the neuron. The neuron is the primary functional unit; this type of cell controls all sensations, movements, thoughts, memories, and feelings through signals that pass through one neuron to another or to the spinal column.

The neuron consists of five parts: the cell body, the dendrites, an axon, the synapse, and an insulating shield (Figure A-4).

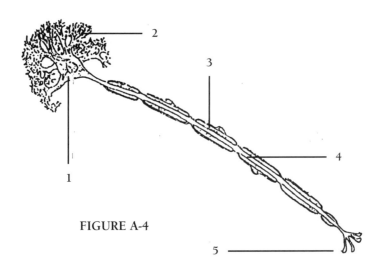

FIGURE A-4

FIGURE A-4

Name	Function
1. Cell body	Holds the nucleus; most of the molecules needed for survival by the neuron are manufactured here.
2. Dendrites	Like the branches of a tree, they protrude out of the cell body and receive messages from other nerve cells. Signals from the dendrites travel through the cell body. They may travel away from the cell down the axon.
3. Axon	Carries signals from the cell body to another neuron, a muscle cell, or cells in one of the organs. May be very short (hair's width) and carry signals in the cortex to another cortex cell. Or they can be quite long and carry signals all the way to the spinal column.
4. Insulating shield	Neurons are usually protected by a group of support cells that wrap around the axon. The insulating shield can include myelin, a fatty molecule which provides further insulation for the axon and assists nerve signals to travel faster and farther.
5. Synapse	The place where a signal passes from the neuron to another cell (see discussion below).

Scientists have been able to learn a great deal about how neurons work by studying the synapse. The synapse is the tiny sac at the end of the neuron. There may be many synapses on each neuron.

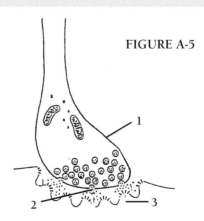

FIGURE A-5

FIGURE A-5

Name	Function
1. Synapse	Stimulated by the signal traveling down the axon.
2. Neurotransmitters	A chemical released by the synapse. They cross the synapse and attach to the receptors of a neighboring cell.
3. Neighboring cell	If it is a neuron, it moves the signal on in the same way. If the neighboring cell is not a neuron, the individual neuron may initiate activity as a transmitter.

The Brain's Transmitters

There is a wide variety of neurotransmitters at work within the neurons which dictate how the cells react under normal conditions. One key neurotransmitter is acetylcholine. It is known as the excitatory neurotransmitter because its primary purpose is to make the cells more excitable. It also governs muscle contractions and causes the glands to secrete hormones. When there is a shortage of acetylcholine in the neuron, it often affects memory formation (as in Alzheimer's disease).

Another critical neurotransmitter is GABA (gamma-aminobutyric acid); this is an inhibitory neurotransmitter. It has the ability to make cells less excitable. This neurotransmitter helps control muscle activity and is an important part of the system involved with sight. With individuals who experience epileptic seizures or tremors, taking a drug(s) containing GABA is often effective in stopping them.

The inhibitory neurotransmitter that constricts blood vessels and brings on sleep is serotonin. Serotonin is also involved with temperature regulation.

Dopamine, another inhibitory neurotransmitter, impacts mood and the control of complex movements. Loss of dopamine activity in some portion of the brain leads to muscle rigidity (as in Parkinson's disease). Behavior disorders are often treated by modifying the action of dopamine in the brain.

With this very basic description of the brain, its functions, and the value of some of the key neurotransmitters, it is easy to understand that there are many places where a brain injury can cause a disruption in everyday activities and normal movements.

Brain Damage

The damage caused by a brain injury most resembles an atomic bomb blast. At the epicenter there is total destruction. As you proceed outward from the center of the blast, the damage is less and less until finally there is no damage.

The core center of the brain injury (damage) represents those cells in the brain that are dead because they have been deprived of oxygen and other necessary nutrients. Once dead, they cannot be revived. In the brain, the area surrounding the core of dead cells is known as the penumbra. The penumbra contains cells that are not working at full capacity, but still have viable neurons that can be reactivated. They are receiving enough O_2 to exist, but not enough to fire electrically. The further you move from the center of the blast, the less damage to the brain. This area (the penumbra) contains the cells of the brain where damage can often be repaired through the use of hyperbaric oxygen therapy (that is, increased oxygen, under pressure, entering into these dormant cells). Although it is not always the case, the penumbra is the area where the SPECT scan will usually show increased activity after hyperbaric oxygen therapy treatments.

The exact location of the damage within the brain, and the extent of the recoverable penumbra, dictate how much a child with cerebral palsy or a traumatic brain injury can recover. As indicated in the illustrations of the brain, the activities affected are determined by the part of the brain that is injured or lacking sufficient oxygen. If a child is to make progress, it will be in the areas of the body managed by the section of the brain where the cells in the penumbra can be revitalized with increased oxygen tension.

Current Research

For hundreds of years, scientists and medical professionals firmly believed that the brain cells an individual was born with were all the brain cells a person would have for a lifetime. Thinking that brain cells would gradually die and never be replaced made it easy to explain why people suffered from memory loss and senility as they got older. No one could prove that this was fact, but neither could anyone prove that it was untrue as there was no way to actually observe brain cells over time.

Equally important to the child who now lives with dormant cells was a discovery made by researchers Beylin, Tanapat, Shors, et al. They proved that cells do live longer and stay stronger if the brain is involved in active learning. While more investigation is necessary, this type of research has provided a strong foundation for understanding the problems of learning disabilities and brain damage. If the brain continues to develop new cells throughout an individual's lifetime, this knowledge may be utilized to help children with brain damage and cerebral palsy. In some ways, this research suggests that in age-related or trauma-related memory loss, the condition is worsened by lack of challenges to the brain. It appears that the brain needs to be presented with new challenges to master in order to maintain thinking and sharpen the memory. This may be part of the reason why children with cerebral palsy and brain injuries continue to improve for an extended period of time after their hyperbaric oxygen treatments have been completed. These children may be using and challenging parts of the brain where cells have been dormant and need to be retrained before progress is noted.

Inasmuch as it has already been proven that hyperbaric oxygen therapy puts more oxygen into the cerebral spinal fluid and plasma and helps increase the flow of blood to the injured cells, this may be yet another reason to immediately place newborns with birth insults into hyperbaric conditions. This may be another step forward in eliminating cerebral palsy in children.

The Impact of Brain Injuries

Brain injuries, regardless of their cause, share common pathophysiologic pathways that result in the destruction of neurons, and to a varying extent, the formation of idling neurons. Knowing how the brain operates makes it easier to understand what happens in serious brain injuries, and how the lack of oxygen can impact the brain's normal functions.

In serious brain injuries, brain damage often occurs because the brain starts to swell from the trauma. This starts a cycle of events that can eventually lead to coma if not rectified quickly. In most instances, the swelling from the initial trauma presses the vulnerable and delicate tissue of the brain against the bony shell of the skull. Unfortunately, the skull does not yield. This impacts the protective fluids that wash over the brain. The increased pressure of the brain pushing against the skull causes the blood supply to the cells to be compromised, and allows for an accumulation of normal wastes that can become toxic when the blood supply is unable to carry the waste away. The cycle continues as the accumulated waste leads to more swelling by further aggravating the swollen brain tissue. HBOT specifically reduces acute and long-term cerebral edema. This is a fact that is supported by the medical profession.

Thus, brain injuries, whether they occur at the time of birth or later in a child's life, regardless of the cause, share common pathophysiological paths. Each injury results in the destruction of neurons, and often includes the formation of idling (dormant) neurons.

This is one of the primary reasons why the sooner a child is treated with HBOT after an injury, the better the prognosis for full recovery. It has now been scientifically proven that HBOT is beneficial in increasing blood flow after an accident, stroke, or other medical insult. Recent studies in other countries have shown that this is particularly true with newborns. In several studies from Europe and South America, published in medical journals, it is stated that children taken from the delivery room to incubators and given compressed air make much better recoveries from difficult births than children who do not receive this treatment.

Many medical professionals who are using hyperbaric oxygen therapy for various injuries, illnesses, and other traumas are convinced that the use of increased oxygen tension may be of more importance to children with learning disabilities and cerebral palsy than was first imagined. It appears that improvements made in motor skills, speaking, and general levels of daily functioning are semi-permanent as a result of HBO therapy. In most cases, only periodic hyperbaric treatments are needed to keep the cells working properly. Equally important to parents is the fact that many children continue to make improvements for several months after hyperbaric oxygen therapy. As noted above, this is consistent with studies by researchers in other countries who have found that using the newly activated cells, over a period of time, brings new levels of learning.

HBOT and the Brain

As stated previously, it has now been scientifically documented that following serious injury, the brain tissue surrounding the injury often contains brain cells that have been stunned, but not killed. Diagnosis, prognosis, and treatment of central nervous system dysfunction requires the ability to differentiate between idling neurons that are viable and living and neurons that are dead. These cells in the penumbra lie in a dormant state between the damaged and the healthy parts of the brain. It is these stunned cells that hyperbaric oxygen therapy can help. HBOT is beneficial to these "at-rest" cells because the increased oxygen tension forces an increased amount of oxygen into the blood plasma.

When oxygen tension is increased, it constricts the normal blood vessels and helps reduce swelling in the brain. Although this at first seems like a contradiction, it is not; the part of the blood where the oxygen is absorbed during increased oxygen tension is different than the part of the blood that normally carries the oxygen in the body. Furthermore, HBOT also forces increased oxygen into the cerebrospinal fluid that surrounds the brain. Working as a team, the plasma and the cerebrospinal fluid can reach areas where the red blood cells that normally carry oxygen cannot penetrate.

Additionally, with the influence of HBOT, oxygen in the capillaries has another advantage over oxygen at standard pressure. Through research studies, HBOT has been proven to push oxygen further into the capillaries of adjacent cells where all life processes take place. Because oxygen is needed for all types of wound healing, the increased oxygen accelerates the healing process of all parts of an injured brain. This evidence of the effectiveness of treating brain damage with HBOT was first publicized in a 1964 report from Dr. V.A. Fasano and his colleagues from the Netherlands. It was further verified through studies conducted in Florida by Dr. Richard Neubauer, and reported in 1985 to the *Lancet*, a British medical journal.

Drs. Astrup, Seisjo, and Symon reported in 1981 that oxygenation is the most critical function of blood flow, and a sudden reduction in oxygen availability is an inevitable consequence of severe ischemia (loss of blood).

Anoxic ischemic encephalopathy (AIE) with severe hypoxia can affect the brain at any age and may result in necrosis and death, but is not always fatal. Patients often exist afterwards in a locked-in syndrome or persistent vegetative coma. These patients are profoundly oxygen deficient and have raised intracranial pressures. Lactic acidosis is also present from anaerobic glycolysis, and there are many other biochemical disturbances, including the generation of oxygen free radical species, which are damaging to neurons. This unfortunate condition has many causes, a few of which are near drowning, near hanging, CO poisoning, cardiac arrest, electrocution, drug overdose, surgical accidents, anesthetic mishaps, and prolonged hypoglycemia. If these patients are treated early with hyperbaric oxygen therapy, the prognosis has been shown to be much more positive.

Worldwide, many patients have been helped, and there is clinical evidence that improved perfusion from reoxygenation has correlated with clinical evidence of benefit, especially with continued therapy. Pressurized oxygen has also been shown to stabilize and repair the layer of cells that stops toxins and many other noxious materials from entering the brain. Labeled the blood-brain barrier, this protective layer of cells is often severely damaged during a head injury.

Conclusion

Possibilities for rehabilitation and recovery depend on the extent and location of irreparable tissue and the surrounding zone of recoverable tissue. With an understanding of brain structure and function, the devastating effects of a brain injury and the necessity of seeking treatment as quickly as possible become readily apparent. Great strides have been made in recent years toward improving our understanding of the brain's capabilities of recovering from trauma, and hyperbaric oxygen therapy has proven to be an important and immensely effective component in the process of restoring function. Current and future research endeavors will lead to promising advances in the treatment modalities that are available to children with cerebral palsy or brain injuries.

THE USE OF HBOT WITH CEREBRAL PALSY AND TRAUMATIC BRAIN INJURIES

*Hyperbaric oxygen provides free molecular oxygen for immediate
metabolic use on a cellular level without the need for energy
exchange, even in the absence of circulation.*
—Edward Teller, Ph.D.

Introduction

The use of oxygen treatments in a hyperbaric chamber is not a new development. The use of increased oxygen tension emerged from the diving industry, and is known as one of the most effective remedies for divers with decompression sickness or more serious diving incidents such as air embolism or a spinal cord insult. As an offshoot of what has been learned from the diving industry about the positive effects of putting pressurized oxygen back into the body's tissues, hyperbaric oxygen therapy has been used for the past few decades as a solution to other medical problems as well.

In the United States, the use of increased oxygen tension delivered in a hyperbaric chamber as a form of medical treatment has gradually increased. As previously discussed, it is widely accepted in the twenty-first century as a remedy for air embolism, carbon monoxide poisoning, and gas gangrene (an infectious type of organism that cannot live in an oxygen-rich environment) as well as other types of damage to the skin, bone, and subcutaneous tissues caused by infection, trauma, or radiation. There is wide acceptance among American doctors for the use of HBOT for the treatment of decompression sickness (the bends) and certain non-healing wounds and infections. As of 2001, the American Medical Association (AMA) and Medicare approved approximately 14 conditions for reimbursement, and treatment for these conditions is routinely reimbursed by most major insurance companies. The list of conditions endorsed by the medical community continues to grow on a regular basis.

The Value of HBOT

It is important to remember that for whatever medical problem HBOT is used, it is not a cure, but rather functions as another system to assist the body's healing process, or as a way of altering the natural history (progression) of certain diseases. It is also known that HBOT aides in removing dead tissue (phagocytosis), scavenging for toxins (free radicals), stimulating collagen production, and growing new blood vessels.

Understanding HBOT

The premise behind HBOT is quite simple. One of the basic components for facilitating the healing process in the body is oxygen. Without adequate oxygen reaching the tissues, cells cannot operate and no wound can heal. By the same principal, many diseases do not improve without properly oxygenated tissue. One of the ways to increase oxygen in the tissues is through pressure. This has been known since the acceptance of Dalton's Law, Charles's Law, and Henry's Law. It has also been proven in clinical studies and is now accepted that an oxygen-rich environment produces a better internal milieu for the growth of new tissue. Sheldon Gottlieb, Ph.D., a leading hyperbaric proponent, has stated that through hyperbarics, oxygen can be delivered to the site of an injury faster, more safely, and in higher concentrations than any other drug.

But what does it mean "to produce a better milieu" for the growth of new tissue? It is easier to understand pressure and its positive effects on neurons if you first become familiar with some of the basic terms used in the gas laws of physics which govern the use of HBOT. It also helps to understand the changes that take place in the body which make HBOT effective. While the physics and physiology of gas laws are quite complicated, the simple explanation presented below provides a sufficient understanding of the effects of HBOT on the body. [For a more detailed explanation, refer to K.K. Jain's, *Textbook of Hyperbaric Medicine*.]

A Simple Explanation of HBOT

The air around us exerts pressure on the body because it has weight. This pressure is about 1 ATM (atmospheric pressure), which is the total weight of air surrounding the earth at sea level.

If you climb up a mountain, however, the pressure on the body and in the body decreases because the air around your body weighs less. The higher you go, the less pressure and the more difficult it becomes to breathe due to less partial pressure of oxygen. People climbing the very highest mountains often develop serious respiratory problems. There is not enough oxygen pressure in the air for the body to receive the proper amount that it needs to function normally.

Conversely, if you dive into the water and go below its surface, pressure in the body increases because the water over your head weighs more the deeper you go. This water pressure, called hydrostatic pressure, increases rapidly because the deeper you go, the more the column of water overhead weighs. This hydrostatic pressure is combined with atmospheric pressure which also exerts its weight on the water. When the two are united, the total pressure (combination of atmospheric and hydrostatic pressures) is called absolute atmospheric pressure. In the context of HBOT, the term given to this absolute pressure is atmospheres absolute (ATA).

Thus, 1.5 ATA is one and a half times the sea-level pressure. When children with cerebral palsy or traumatic head injuries breathe pure oxygen at 1.25 - 1.5 ATA, this added pressure forces more oxygen into the body's tissues even in areas of compromised circulation, whereas breathing pure oxygen at sea level cannot achieve the same effect.

In hyperbaric oxygen therapy, all of the body is affected, but no part more so than the brain, a remarkable organ that has the ability to change injured and non-injured neurons in a positive direction. The air that we normally breathe is about 21% oxygen; the rest is nitrogen and other inert components. In hyperbaric oxygen therapy, the patient breathes 100% oxygen under increased pressure, and the concentration of oxygen normally dissolved in the blood plasma is raised many times above normal. In addition to the brain cells and blood, all body fluids, including the lymph and cerebrospinal fluid, are infused with the healing benefits of this molecular oxygen. The pressurized oxygen can also reach bone tissue, enhance white blood cell function, and promote the formation of new capillaries and peripheral blood vessels. All of these powerful improvements make the body use all of its parts more effectively and efficiently, and the outcome for improved prognosis of any injury or brain damage may rise dramatically.

The Impact of Hypoxia (Reduced Oxygen)

One of the major causes of cerebral palsy is hypoxia occurring before, at, or just after birth. While the term "hypoxia" means a reduced supply of oxygen in the cells of the organism, the term "anoxia" usually indicates a total lack of oxygen. According to K.K. Jain, it is difficult to define hypoxia precisely, but it can best be described as a state in which the "aerobic metabolism is reduced by the fall of PO_2 within the mitochondria." Therefore, although any part of the body can be affected by this lack of oxygen in the cells, the effects are most marked on the cells of the nervous system for the following reasons:

the brain has unusually high and constant energy requirements;

the brain cannot store much oxygen; and

neurons have a poor capacity to recover after anoxia/hypoxia.

HBOT as a Medical Therapy

Simply defined, hyperbaric oxygen therapy is a medical treatment that uses pure oxygen at increased ambient pressure to speed and enhance the body's natural ability to heal. In cases of cerebral palsy and brain traumas, the brain tissue is revived and can assist the child in restoring those functions that have been lost or compromised. It is interesting to note that the recovery of the child's motor and intellectual functions often continues long after the treatments have ended. The brain cells that have been dormant need to re-learn (or, perhaps, learn for the first time) the functions for which they are responsible.

Inasmuch as the brain consumes 20% of the oxygen in the body even though it makes up only 2% of the weight, it is easy to see why lack of oxygen in the brain cells has such a dramatic effect on the body. The brain also receives 15% of the cardiac output even though it does not perform any physical work. Lack of oxygen is devastating to a child's brain. In cases of cerebral palsy and brain injury, the goal is to "jump-start" the dormant brain cells with HBOT by providing adequate oxygen to create a better internal environment and encourage optimal development. In some cases, damaged neurons can be recovered up to 12 - 14 years after an injury occurs. Thus, many types of brain insults, including pediatric stroke, coma, and even children with autism have been successfully treated through the use of HBOT.

Ongoing Research

Further study, particularly controlled tests, will be necessary to determine exactly how and to what extent HBOT can be used on brain injuries other than cerebral palsy and brain trauma. Hyperbaric physicians are collaborating on an international level to investigate the helpful effects of HBOT on multiple health problems. Within the past few years, for example, the Space and Underwater Research Group of the World Federation of Neurology has sanctioned a protocol for the use of HBOT within the first four hours of stroke, with or without clot-dissolving drugs. Previous data has indicated that early intervention is also extremely important in traumatic brain injury. Reduction in mortality and morbidity has been reported as high as 40% in literature from Wassmann and Holbach as well as Rockswold. Many hyperbaric physicians have been successfully treating stroke victims since the early 1980s. In addition, physicians in the U.S. and abroad have increasing opportunities to experience first-hand the benefits of HBOT on multiple sclerosis, age-related macular degeneration, acquired immune deficiency syndrome (AIDS), Lyme disease, cerebral palsy, and brain injuries.

Studies from around the world are currently yielding impressive results demonstrating that reactivating dormant brain cells with HBOT can have positive effects on many types of pediatric brain injuries. More importantly, there are compelling reports suggesting that hyperbaric oxygenation should be administered as soon as possible in cases of cerebral palsy and the brain-injured child to achieve the maximum effect. One study, reported in 1992, found that HBO treatment administered soon after an acute head injury has the ability to reduce mortality by more than 40%. At the same time, it has been discovered that in some cases, damaged neurons can be recovered several years after an injury occurs. HBOT can thus be considered as a viable treatment modality for a wide range of individuals.

Researchers are also investigating possibilities for administering HBOT in prenatal and immediate postnatal cases. Presently, doctors in Sicily (Sparacia, et al.) are conducting tests based on a study that took place in Russia more than 15 years ago. In the Russian study, researchers used HBOT to treat acute hypoxia in labor and fetal growth delay due to placental insufficiency. They placed the newly delivered infant in a chamber with 100% oxygen under pressure. Sparacia, among others, believes that HBOT is irreplaceable in improving both placental blood flow and oxygen diffusion at the cellular level (in the womb). This study indicates that HBOT for maternal causes prior to the gestation period, hypochromic or hemolytic anemia, uterine pathology involving a reduction of the placental implantation surface, abnormalities in various organs, any cyanogen, and pulmonary lesions, as well as hypertensive preeclampsia syndrome and placental alterations, reduce the exchange function of fetus/placenta. It will be beneficial for high-risk pregnancies if further studies prove that the fetus can be treated with HBO in the womb.

Progress continues to be made. With these advances in research, the outlook is improving for the medical profession to recognize the value of HBOT for children with cerebral palsy and other neurological conditions. For information on a number of other studies currently taking place concerning the effects of HBOT on children with cerebral palsy, refer to Chapter 10.

Conclusion

It has been established that HBOT is a method of administering pure oxygen to a patient at greater than atmospheric pressure with the purpose of improving or correcting certain neurological conditions. Success of hyperbaric oxygen therapy in any given case is dependent upon the location and extent of the irreparable damage and the location and extent of the potentially recoverable areas in the brain, overall physical condition, and/or severity of the patient's injury. While not necessarily a cure, hyperbaric oxygen treatments offer the best chance of recovery for patients suffering from a variety of medical conditions. When administered properly by trained medical personnel under the supervision of an experienced hyperbaric physician, HBOT causes no pain or discomfort and is completely non-invasive. At the same time, the caregiver is encouraged to fully investigate any hyperbaric center before using it to treat a child with cerebral palsy or a traumatic brain injury.

When children with cerebral palsy or brain injuries are treated at an early age, not only can repair of the damaged areas be effected, but a more appropriate environment for the continued development and encouragement of the growing brain can be established.

CONTROLLING SEIZURES IN CEREBRAL PALSY AND BRAIN INSULTS

*If hyperbaric oxygenation proves to help reduce seizures
in children with cerebral palsy, thousands of children will lead
a far more normal life with less medication.*

—Ed Nemeth
Rebecca's father

Introduction

One of the most debilitating conditions for many children with cerebral palsy, especially those with high muscle tone, is seizures. It is suspected that about 50% of children with cerebral palsy have some degree or type of seizures. Children who have quadriplegic or hemiplegic types of cerebral palsy are the most likely to have serious seizures.

The exact cause of seizures may differ slightly from child to child, but in general, the cause is related to the electrical changes in the brain which make movement, speech, thought, and bodily functions possible. Under normal circumstances, nerve transmission in the brain occurs without any problems, and the average person gives little thought to how the smooth flow of electrical activity occurs or what happens when it is disrupted. Both normal and abnormal brain cells can sometimes function abnormally, but for many children with cerebral palsy it happens with regularity. When there is abnormal function in the brain, the neurons generate uncoordinated electrical charges that can spread to one group of muscles or throughout the body. When this happens, the body reacts, sometimes violently and sometimes with only a twitch of the face. Whatever the degree of the impact on the body, the event is classified as a seizure.

Types of Seizures

For many years, seizures were referred to as petit mal and grand mal. These two terms have been further defined as absence (petit mal) and tonic-clonic (grand mal), or as generalized onset (tonic-clonic) and focal or partial.

Absence (petit mal) seizures cause a brief, abrupt loss of consciousness (lasting a few seconds) followed by a rapid, complete recovery. It appears that in an absence seizure, the part of the brain that makes individuals "aware" temporarily loses communication with the brain cortex. This type of seizure is said to be "non-convulsive"; the child may sit and stare or have repetitive eye blinking. This is sometimes referred to as a typical petit mal seizure. Realistically, this type of seizure may involve minor twitching (often almost unnoticed) that disrupts the child's attention momentarily and brings about temporary diminished muscle tone. It often causes the child to lose eye contact as well, which further diminishes the ability to observe non-verbal aspects of life that are critical to learning. This includes but certainly is not limited to focusing on facial expressions, body language, and other subtle means of learning. If these signs are not detected, children are often accused of "not paying attention" to what they are being told. The caregiver is aware that the child seems to lose focus, but often does not realize what is happening. Medically, these sudden, instantaneous changes are referred to as "startle" seizures.

In a complex partial seizure, the child may hallucinate, stagger, perform automatic and purposeless movements, or experience confusion or impaired consciousness. For the most part, only one part of the body will be impacted initially, but the seizure may become more generalized.

The more common form of seizure that children with cerebral palsy have is the tonic-clonic. The word "tonic" means to stiffen and "clonic" means to jerk. In the tonic phase, muscles throughout the body may stiffen briefly, and then the child will fall to the floor unconscious. In the clonic phase, there are major spasms that can last for one to several minutes or even hours wherein the extremities jerk.

General-onset or tonic-clonic are convulsive seizures; they are often referred to as epilepsy if they are repetitive and/or severe. The term epilepsy refers to recurrent, unprovoked seizures of any type. General-onset seizures start in one part of the brain, but quickly spread to other parts. This is what causes muscle twitching, convulsions, salivating, rigidity, or other types of unnatural movement. These spasms gradually become slower and less intense until they pass entirely. During the intense part of the seizure, however, the child is unable to breathe correctly, may lose control of the bladder, and often seems blue around the lips. The child may even cry out during the seizure or lose consciousness. The child will wake up dazed, confused, and very tired. On rare occasions, such seizures can be fatal.

These different types of seizures are quite different in strength and length, but all interrupt the cognitive learning process and disrupt alertness for the duration of the seizure.

Seizures can be further classified as partial or generalized. In partial seizures, only one side of the body is affected because only one side of the brain is receiving inappropriate electrical discharges. In the generalized type, both sides of the brain are impacted and reacting abnormally, so both sides of the body are affected.

There is a another type of seizure known as the febrile seizure. Most often, febrile seizures are convulsions triggered by a high fever in infants or small children. During a febrile seizure, a child will typically lose consciousness and begin to shake, with limbs on both sides of the body being involved. Occasionally, a child will twitch or become rigid in only one part of the body. In most children, this type of seizure will last from a few seconds to a few minutes, but they have been known to last for 15 minutes or more. The vast majority of febrile seizures are harmless and do not cause brain damage, but for children who have a long series of this type of seizure, there is a chance that they will develop cerebral palsy, delayed development, or other type of neurological problem.

Another, more serious type of seizure in infants is infantile myoclonic seizures (infantile seizures). This type of seizure lasts only seconds, but may happen many times a day. In this type of seizure, there are sudden, brief, involuntary muscle contractions that involve one or many of the muscle groups. The most common movements are drooping of the head and flexing of the body, legs, and arms; this type of seizure is sometimes referred to as a jackknife seizure.

One of the most dangerous seizures is the atonic (akinetic) seizure. In this type of seizure, there is an overall sudden loss of body tone. This type of seizure, which occurs with little, if any, warning, may cause the child to fall and be hurt. For this reason, many children with this type of seizure wear helmets to protect their heads against such falls.

Areas in the Brain Where Seizures Occur

Certain parts of the brain are more likely to be the primary location of seizures than other parts. The motor cortex (the part of the brain responsible for the start of movement in the body) and the temporal lobes (specifically the hippocampus, the part of the inner brain which is responsible for memory) are the two brain sections that seem to be most often affected. It is thought that the motor cortex and the temporal lobes are especially sensitive to situations that cause abnormal electrical transmission. These include but are not limited to decreased oxygen levels, infections, and metabolic changes. Clinical studies have shown that there are many other types of brain abnormalities that can be responsible for producing seizure activity as well, but the three listed here are the most common.

What Causes a Seizure?

To understand how the process of electricity works within a neuron, the illustration of a neuron with its various components is provided below. Understanding how the neuron functions makes it much easier to understand how and why a seizure occurs.

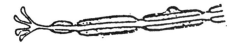

As shown in the illustration, the neuron resembles a tube that has an inner section and an outer coating. The compositions of the inner and outer cells are quite different. The inner cell section has a much higher concentration of potassium than does the outer wall (membrane), while the outer membrane has a much higher concentration of sodium than does the inner part. In the normal resting state of a neuron, membrane pumps are constantly at work to maintain each ion (sodium and potassium) in the proper area until it is needed. When a neuron is needed to transmit a signal, these ions (salts) move along the neuron from one end to another, rather like a wave going to shore. When the signal reaches the end of the neuron (known as the synapse), the signal is transferred to the adjoining cell either by a direct extension of this process or by releasing a neurotransmitter, a special type of chemical.

There are two primary types of neurotransmitter. The type that causes cell-to-cell communication is known as an "excitatory" neurotransmitter. The type that is able to slow down or stop cell-to-cell communication is called an "inhibitory" transmitter. Sometimes over-activity of excitatory neurotransmitter or under-activity of inhibitory neurotransmitter will set off seizures because they cause an uncoordinated flow of electrical activity in the brain.

To put it more simply, neurons resemble small telephone wires running through the brain. These tiny wires send signals to different parts of the brain; this is how we think and move. When these signals are interrupted (i.e., made to go too fast or too slow), it causes an uneven flow of activity. This makes for changes in the biochemistry of the brain and disrupts communication between the cells. Thus, when a person has a seizure, it is because the neurons in the brain are either firing when they should not or are not firing when they should. There can be an uncontrolled discharge that affects several parts of the brain and then spreads to both sides of the body, or there might be an impact on only one part of the brain that affects a specific part of the body.

Recurrent or prolonged seizures (20 - 30 minutes) can permanently damage neurons. When a seizure, no matter what its severity, occurs on a regular basis and is unprovoked, the medical term is epilepsy. If a seizure of any type is intense, frequent, or prolonged, the child is most often given medication to reduce both the severity and the frequency of seizures.

Treatment of Cerebral Palsy

Cerebral palsy cannot, at this time, be cured, but when neurological problems are managed efficiently, the child will have a better chance of leading a near-normal life. There appears to be no treatment that works for all children; for this reason, caregivers must work with physicians, therapists, and other healthcare professionals, including nutritionists and chiropractors, to develop a plan that works best for the individual child. Sometimes this plan includes drugs to control seizures and muscle spasms, special braces to compensate for muscle imbalance, surgery, or mechanical aids, such as computerized boards, to assist with speaking.

The members of a treatment team will most often include one or more of the following: a pediatrician, a pediatric neurologist or pediatric physiatrist, an orthopedic doctor, a physical therapist, an occupational therapist, a speech and language pathologist, and a social worker to help the family find the correct educational center or resource as well as a psychologist and education professionals. This group of individuals is most often able to manage the conditions of the child, but none of these services are meant to solve the entire problem.

Although each of these professionals can contribute to a better lifestyle for the child, the caregivers are the key members of the team. The caregivers not only need to decide which of the professional team members to use, but also must be closely involved in all steps of planning, decision-making, and treatments. Often, the caregiver actually does most of the therapy work with the child on a daily basis after a plan has been established. The caregiver is the primary person involved in "patterning" if it is incorporated into the child's therapy. Patterning is a controversial, relatively new therapy in which a sequence of movements is used to guide the child with movement problems. The child is taught to pull him- or herself erect and then to crawl, as these movements are considered essential to learning to walk. There is also behavioral therapy that challenges a child to overcome specific permanent handicaps by using psychological theory and techniques that complement physical, speech, or occupational therapies.

At this time, therapy, whether for movement, speech, or living skills, is the primary treatment for cerebral palsy. The therapist merely serves as the coach to assist the caregiver in understanding the strategies and theories behind each form of therapy.

These therapies are frequently combined with drug therapy. The types of drugs given to children with cerebral palsy are usually based on the types of seizures they experience. Of course, no single drug controls all types of seizures or helps all children. Different children, even with the same type of seizures, may do better on different medications. In some cases, it is necessary to give a combination of drugs in order to achieve the best conditions for living and learning. Medications most often used in the past few years for controlling seizures are Diazepam, Lannietal, and Depakote. There are also medications to control spasticity.

Diazepam (Valium) is used as a general relaxant of the brain and body; baclofen blocks signals sent from the brain to contract the muscles; and dantrolene (a muscle relaxant) reduces the process of muscle contractions. Lamictal and Depakote are also anti-seizure medications. Although the value of these specific drugs for long-term control of spasticity has not yet been fully proven clinically, it is known that these drugs help many children on a short-term basis. Unfortunately, their long-term effect on the developing nervous system is not fully understood, and in some children, the drugs cause dry mouth and drowsiness to such a high degree that the benefits are questionable. At times, the treatment may be worse than the condition for certain children.

Other drugs, such as those belonging to a group of chemicals called anticholinergics, are also used to help reduce abnormal movements. This group of anticholinergics, including Trihexyphenidyl, Benztropine, and Procyclidine Hydrochloride, work by reducing the activity of acetylcholine, one of the body's chemicals that helps some brain cells communicate and triggers muscle contractions.

Other times, a botulism toxin injection may be administered directly into the muscle to reduce spasticity, or surgery may be performed to ease severe contractures. Again, there are consequences; the botulism injection is only a temporary measure, and the surgery is often followed by months of recovery. Additionally, it must be determined exactly which muscle is causing the contracting problem or the problem could be exacerbated.

Conclusion

Reducing seizures, stopping seizures entirely, and/or reducing the need for seizure medication is one of the areas where hyperbaric oxygen therapy (HBOT) has been most successful. The increased oxygen tension is able to penetrate the tissues that are dormant to help regulate erratic brain activity. Increased oxygen pressure assists the small electrical impulses to act in a normal, productive manner to send smooth, coordinated messages to the rest of the body. Inasmuch as cerebral palsy is caused by the misfiring or slow firing of the electrical impulses in the brain, putting extra oxygen into the cells is a logical way to improve the function of damaged parts of the brain.

SPECT SCANS:
THE DIAGNOSTIC
EVALUATOR

*Diagnostic imaging plays an important role in diagnosis of
diseases of the central nervous system. It is even more important in
assessing the effects of HBO on hypoxic/ischemic lesions of the brain.*
—K.K. Jain

Introduction

The SPECT (single-photon emission-computed tomography) scan is
one of the methods most frequently used to measure the active neurons
in the brain and to discover cells in the penumbra that may be inactive,
but alive. This is technically referred to as functional brain imaging.
"Functional brain imaging refers to that set of techniques used to derive
images reflecting biochemical, physiologic, or electrical properties of the
central nervous system (CNS)."

There are actually two systems used for functional brain imaging:
positron emission tomography (PET) and SPECT. A SPECT scan is most
often used for children with cerebral palsy and brain injuries because it
is the most widely available and most widely applicable measure of neuron behavior. Although PET provides higher resolution tomographic
images of brain function, this difference between PET and SPECT is not
critical; for clinical applications, the differences in resolution are incon-
sequential. SPECT, however, is generally reimbursable by most insurers
while PET has a very limited coverage for cerebral palsy and the brain-
injured child.

This chapter provides a comprehensive overview of SPECT as well as
a detailed discussion of procedures, the gamma camera, and the information revealed by using the SPECT scan.

It should be noted that there were significant changes in functional brain imaging as new discoveries were made between 1995 and 2000. For example, there are now non-camera-based and camera-based systems, with the camera-based system being the one most frequently used in academic or medical settings. It is likely that more changes will take place in the next few years as well. Past changes include improvements in instruments, time required to conduct the test, and the radiopharmaceuticals used as radio tracers, but the differences do not detract from the images the original SPECT scanners produced. For this reason, the exact configuration or the age of the SPECT camera used is not critical when evaluating the effectiveness of a hyperbaric center or its gamma camera.

What is a SPECT Scan?

Single photon emission computed tomography (SPECT) scanning is a fairly new, advanced, diagnostic nuclear medical imaging procedure that provides a "cross section" image of the body similar to those generated by computerized tomography (CT), also known as computerized axial tomography (CAT). Its primary purpose is to determine blood flow in the various organs of the body. It is particularly beneficial in the study of the brain. Unlike MRI or CAT scans, whose purpose is to show the anatomy of the body, SPECT scans show actual body functions, including brain function. An infinitesimal amount of a short-lived radioactive tracer is injected into an individual's bloodstream through the arm or any vein. It releases energy impulses which are then identified by the sensitive detectors of the SPECT scanner. The radioisotope used for tracing brains has the ability to cross the blood-brain barrier, which allows the doctor to determine how blood is distributed through different parts of the brain and to visualize brain metabolism. The scans produced by the gamma camera give the doctor the means to distinguish between dead and living cells, to determine the effects of pre and post HBO treatments, and to make a better diagnosis of the patient's actual condition.

A SPECT scan is a non-confining, painless procedure. The patient lies on a gurney that is rolled into the middle of the SPECT scan camera. The patient lies quietly on the gurney with his or her head in a steady position for 30 - 40 minutes. During this time, the gamma camera rotates (circles) around the head as it picks up impulses, and takes a 360° image of the brain. This data (in photo form) is transferred to a special computer that compiles a photo-picture (digital image) of the brain in three planes. These digital images are examined and evaluated by the hyperbaric and nuclear physicians to determine brain function in much the same way as another specialist might use an x-ray, sonogram, or MRI to determine the condition of a specific part or organ of the body.

At times, it is conducive to good imaging to give younger or spastic children a small amount of sedative to help them remain still during the photo-taking process. The most common products used to sedate children during SPECT scanning are oral chloral hydrate and sodium Butisol, injectable Versed or Valium, or Valium suppositories. The dose is calculated according to the child's weight so that the sedation will pass off quickly and safely. This usually takes place within an hour after the scan is performed.

The initial scan of the brain gives a baseline report of its function. This is critical in making a correct diagnosis of the progress and value of hyperbaric oxygen therapy. It is usually imperative that there be areas of the brain which show the ability to recover through the use of increased oxygen tension. If no idling brain cells are located, HBOT may not be helpful. There have been instances, however, when significant improvement has taken place in a patient in spite of the absence of visible recoverable neurons. Cases such as these may be evidence of the brain's capacity for plasticity. This is the ability of one part of the brain to take over for another part, and is the basis of neuro-rehabilitation.

Preparation for the SPECT Scan

Visualizing brain function requires the presence of a "tracer" that can be "photographed" from various angles. A diffusible tracer is one that passes through the circulation without engaging in metabolism. There are several types of radiotracers that can be used, but each type utilizes a small radioisotope which emits discernable photon impulses. Two of the radiotracers most commonly used are Technetium 99 HMPAO–Ceretec or Technitium 99m E.C.D. (Neurolite). Only a small amount of this radiotracer material, injected into the bloodstream, is required for the process to be effective. This injection is given to the patient about 20 - 40 minutes before the SPECT scan actually takes place to give the tracer time to circulate through the bloodstream to all parts of the body, including the brain. The radiotracer then disintegrates and is naturally filtered from the body within an hour or so without having any metabolic effect.

How the Scan Measures Brain Function

The tracer is injected into the bloodstream, and then crosses the blood-brain barrier to circulate into deep regions of the brain. This allows the gamma camera to pinpoint the position and energy of photon impulses as the radiotracer disintegrates. The tracer circulates though living brain tissue, including areas that are normal and areas that are damaged but salvageable. In this way, sequential (follow-up) SPECT scans can easily distinguish between living (but dormant) and dead (necrotic) tissue. SPECT performed pre and post HBOT can prove that there are recoverable brain cells. These are referred to in this book as dormant or idling neurons, but the proper name for recoverable brain tissue is the ischemic penumbra.

K.K. Jain explains that for most purposes, the best and most expedient method to assess the HBO potential and endpoint of treatment is SPECT brain imaging on a high resolution camera. SPECT scans completed before and after HBOT at any point in the treatment process may help identify its potential for success.

Technically, the gamma camera detects the position and energy of photon impulses emitted from the decaying tracer. The image is reconstructed into tomographic slices, with a color scale assigned in proportion to the strength of the signal. Thus, SPECT scans measure the brain's uptake of the minute amounts of radiotracer during the course of its normal functioning. SPECT scan images may also be produced in black and white. In these cases, there is an inverse scale describing degrees of function. Rather, areas that appear white indicate normally functioning brain cells, while dark areas indicate non-functioning but potentially recoverable brain cells.

There is no single gamma camera or tracer isotope that is universally used in the United States. It is a matter of preference for the hyperbaric center or the physician. For the same reasons that all medical centers do not use the same brand or style of equipment, there are several types of SPECT scanning equipment as well.

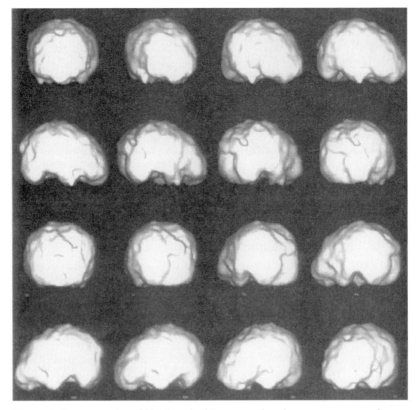

Figure 1 shows a series of black and white scans that demonstrate normal brain function.

Some Remarkable Case Studies

Pre Scan

The pre scan in Figure 2 is of a three-year-old male near-drowning victim. The patient presented in a persistent vegetative state with severe spasticity on the left and hypermobility of the right leg. The family was told that the child was blind, and it was necessary to feed him using a PEG tube. Initial SPECT scans showed an extensive and symmetric deficiency throughout the frontal, temporal, parietal, and occipital lobes. Areas that appear white indicate oxygen-rich neurons that are actively functioning. Dark areas indicate that parts of the brain that are idling, but not receiving enough oxygen to function normally.

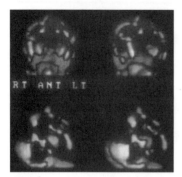 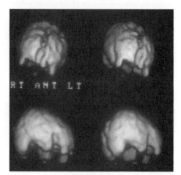

Initial   One year and three months later

FIGURE 2 Pre and Post Scans

This pre-treatment scan indicated large areas of hypoperfusion or lack of oxygen that could recoverable; these cells were merely in an electrically inactive or idling state. The SPECT scan helped the doctor to determine that this child would, in all probability, benefit from hyperbaric oxygen therapy.

Post Scan

The post scan in Figure 2 is the same child taken one year and three months after he began hyperbaric oxygen treatments. The white area in this "after" scan indicates recovered brain cells and reactivated neurons surrounding the severely damaged and oxygen-deficient areas of the brain. There is increased brain activity and blood flow.

After three treatments with HBO, the patient was more mobile, tried to use his vocal cords, and "acted up" when angry. The patient began crying real tears after 16 treatments. After 26 treatments, the patient was smiling, more alert, laughing, crying, sleeping better, and laughing while dreaming. Following 34 treatments, the patient became increasingly alert and made more eye contact—certainly not blind. To date, the patient has received 154 treatments and now sees clearly, is speaking bilingually, standing and taking a few steps, and takes all food by mouth.

This child advanced from the grave prediction of his pediatric neurologist—who said his outlook for recovery was "zero"—to a much better life expectancy. He is able to attend preschool, play chase-and-tumble games with his older brother, and is a very active, nearly normal four-year-old.

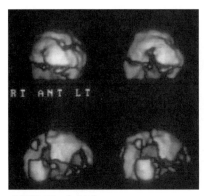 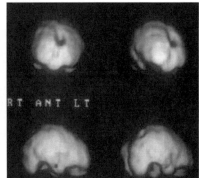

CASE GS - Initial   CASE GS - One month later

Case GS

An 8 1/2 year-old female in MVA suffered a closed head injury eleven months prior. The patient was comatose for 4 months. Improvement began about 6 months. The patient was aphasic, could understand, but not verbalize. There was ataxia and dysarthia. The patient had marked spasticity and crossed legs and feet while walking, which was worse on the left. No control of left arm was noted. Following 90 hyperbaric oxygen treatments, there was substantial improvement. She was able to stand with assistance. Her speech was louder and her verbalization increased. Both range of motion and spasticity improved. She was much more aware, able to sit up straight, and follow commands. She became very aware, comprehension was now normal and she processes information well. She was now able to do back extension on command and to move all extremities on command. She was able to do push-ups from a sitting position. She was able to stand straight with the help of bars. She was able to throw a kiss. The outlook became tremendously improved and the level of care greatly diminished.

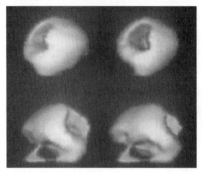 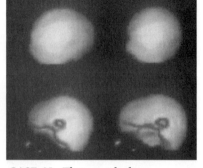

CASE AI - Initial   **CASE AI - Three weeks later**

Case AI

This patient is a three-year-old girl born 1 pound 11 ounces at 26 weeks gestation by emergency C-section due to placenta previa. Cerebral plasy developed and was manifest by severe four extremity spasticity, hyper reflexia, clonus, microcephaly, developmental delay and retinopathy of prematurity. Basline SPECT pre HBOT showed hypoperfusion in the basal ganglia, thalami and occipital lobes with simultaneous improvement in alertness, verbal and gross motor skills, sleep, vision, cognition, and a decrease in spasticity.

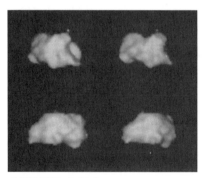 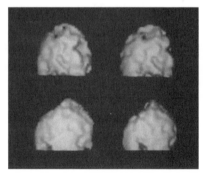

CASE EW - Initial   **CASE EW - One month later**

Case EW

A three-year-old white male who suffered perinatal hypoxic ischemic encephalopathy with renal failure acute tubular necrosis, thrombocytopenia, sepsis, respiratory insuffiency, hypovolemia and apnea related seizure disorder. CT scan showed progressive cortical atrophy. It is remarkable that this patient survived. The patient received 21 treatments of HBO and is now able to sit up, hold a cup for the first time and is more attentive. He is much more alert, makes new vocal sounds, is more aware of his surroundings, and is beginning to grab at everything. These changes parallel SPECT scan imprint.

Future SPECT Scans

The baseline SPECT scan is compared with sequential SPECT scans (performed post HBOT). These sequential imaging studies can clearly indicate whether parts of the brain are functioning more effectively. In children with cerebral palsy, the second SPECT scan is usually given toward the end of the first course of treatments so that changes can be discussed with the caregiver and a decision made about future treatments.

Correlation of SPECT to Success Rate of HBOT

Although HBOT may not improve every child with cerebral palsy or a traumatic brain injury, in about 80 - 90% of the cases, improved SPECT scans correlate to improvements in the patient's physical condition. In particular, positive changes are often seen in motor functions, from the complex muscle contractions involved in swallowing to increased ability to maintain balance, stand, and walk.

Ownership of SPECT Scans

Hyperbaric centers have different policies about the SPECT scan, but in some instances copies of the scans are given to the child's caregiver for review by the child's primary physician and/or care-giving team. Because the prescribed dose (total number of treatments and pressure) varies from patient to patient, the timing of the SPECT scans varies as well. For the most part, the costs of the pre and periodic post SPECT scans are covered by major insurance company policies.

Ongoing Improvement

In children with cerebral palsy, caregivers often report that the child continues to improve long after the initial HBOT has stopped. When there is no other change in the child's treatment regimen, most care-givers conclude that the improvements are the result of HBOT. For this reason, they often return for additional treatments when they see no fur-ther improvement in the child's daily functioning. This has proven to be valuable in many children. The HBO treatments that are helping children with cerebral palsy satisfy the second cardinal rule of medicine: treat until the patient no longer benefits from treatment. In many instances, improvement following HBOT may be observed in children with acute brain insults on the first or second treatment, and in other children, improvement may come after the treatments are concluded.

Conclusion

The single photon emission computed tomography (SPECT) scan is becoming more readily available, and the computer-assisted evaluation methods are continually improving. This will make the use of this system for evaluating the activity of the brain more accessible to the general public, probably at a reduced cost. It is easy to use with children and is safe and harmless. Radiopharmaceuticals (radiotracers) provide a way to "photograph" the brain and then pass out of the body after they have been used to document blood flow, metabolism, or brain functions. While the initial SPECT provides the baseline report of the functioning of the brain, sequential imaging studies tell the effects of HBO treatments.

The use of SPECT scans provides proof that HBOT improves blood flow and function to areas of the brain that were not actively operating during the pre-treatment scan. The periodic use of the SPECT scan during and after HBO treatments provides concrete evidence that positive changes in the brain are continuing to take place and remaining in place even after several months.

J. Michael Uszler, M.D., Director of the Nuclear Medicine Department at Santa Monica UCLA (University of California Los Angeles), is one of the leading specialists in the use of the SPECT scan. He has stated, "I have seen over one hundred patients, children and adults, with serious brain injuries who have had baseline SPECT scans, hyperbaric oxygenation treatment, then repeat SPECT scans. There is a close correlation between the positive changes in SPECT scans and clinical status. In fact, at times, the clinical results have been surprising. Utilizing the same patient as 'his or her own control,' with hyperbaric oxygenation as the only variable, scientifically documents the positive effect of this therapy."

At this time, hyperbaric oxygen therapy is seldom given in isolation. It is most often administered in conjunction with ongoing speech, occupational, and physical therapies. These other therapies are continued while the child receives HBO treatments.

REBECCA'S STORY:
ONE CHILD'S JOURNEY
(Written by her Daddy, Ed Nemeth)

*"Every journey starts with a single step. If we could begin
our journey again, we would begin it on the footing of this book."*
— DENISE AND ED NEMETH

My wife, Denise, and I had a perfect life planned for us and our soon-to-be-born child. We had established ourselves financially and planned out every aspect of caring for our, at that time, healthy unborn child, Rebecca.

But no amount of preparation prepared us for the tragedy that struck: Rebecca "died" at birth for 35 minutes and was on life support for the first six days of her life, virtually brain dead.

We were terrified of Rebecca eventually dying "by herself," so we made the decision to remove her from life support so that she could die in our arms with all of our love surrounding her. We dressed Rebecca in her prettiest outfit, put a bow in her hair, and went into a private room with a nurse. We were fully aware of the tragic finality of this decision. Rebecca stopped breathing twice in the first ten minutes. The second time it happened, the nurse thought she had passed. As we cried for our lost baby, our tears fell on her beautiful face and touched her soul. Somehow, Rebecca caught her breath, and two hours later was breathing regularly with good color.

At 10:00 p.m., we put her to bed and kissed her good night. At that moment, Rebecca literally opened her eyes and began to move her arms and legs, and she cried. Of course, we were ecstatic. But her miracle was so extreme and so complete, we did not know that a true miracle had occurred.

The doctors, of course, thought we were mistaken. They told us she would not survive. When she continued to survive, they said she could not see. When it became apparent that she could see, they thought she would be a vegetable. When Rebecca decided she did not like peas and carrots, we knew she could think. It soon became obvious that she was a very bright young lady, with a sparkling personality and a heart warming smile. She also was severely afflicted with cerebral palsy.

This was our initiation into the inability of otherwise excellent physicians to discern who Rebecca was and how we should manage her medical care. In fairness to all the medical community who tried to help us, Rebecca's survival was completely unexplainable. And while she was very bright, there was no question about the extent of her brain injuries. In fact, Rebecca was one of the most severely afflicted cerebral palsy children in our immediate medical community.

At first, our greatest challenge was to obtain factual information about the exact nature of Rebecca's injuries and to learn about the medical treatments that were available to help her. Preconceptions and biases delayed our journey from the beginning. Thus, we began our long journey in search of this book.

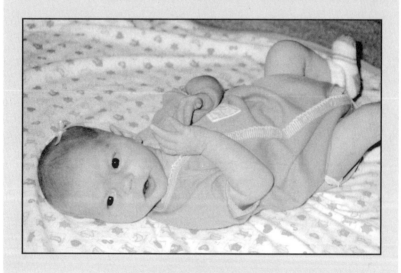

While Rebecca was in the neo-intensive care unit of the hospital, her mother and I instinctively began helping Rebecca move her arms and legs. We wanted to keep them from becoming stiff. We believed we could keep Rebecca from developing contractures by keeping her limbs moving and flexible. (Of course, the NICU physical therapist was not allowed to spend time with us because the doctors did not think Rebecca would live. In fact, they continued to say she would not live.)

Finally, when the physical therapist noticed that we were not smart enough to believe what the medical experts told us, she gave us physical therapy instructions. As a result of this early work, and our efforts that continued throughout her life, Rebecca has never had a problem with contractures and all of the related disabilities.

(It is part of the theorem that the earlier you start treatment, the more often the results are favorable.)

When Rebecca was ready to leave the neo-intensive care unit, we were primarily on our own. We immediately began searching for information about cerebral palsy, physical therapies, and answers we needed to other medical questions. At first, we bought a number of excellent books. They were full of definitions, but contained very little in the way of care management insights.

At the same time, we were searching for the best neurologist in the United States. That's how we met Dr. William Mobley of the UCSF Medical Center. We were very lucky; Dr. Mobley not only knew Rebecca's neurologist, Dr. Asaikar, but thought the world of him. This was a great help to us in organizing Rebecca's care and making certain we did everything we could to help her. Not everyone is so lucky to have two such wonderful doctors caring for their child. Thus, we had more information and understanding of the problem than most parents.

In spite of all they could tell us, however, we still had great difficulty pulling together all of the information we required to fully help Rebecca develop.

Several times during the first three years of her life, we were fully responsible for keeping her alive until we could get to an emergency room. Knowing infant cardio pulmonary resuscitation (CPR) was not at option for us; it was a necessity.

We worked with Rebecca on every aspect of her development using every technique we could learn about. She flourished under the various physical therapies we tried and she developed well, with no contractures and good flexibility.

But while Rebecca was developing far better than many other children who had far less injuries and damage, she hit a stubborn plateau. Her greatest challenge, gaining head control, continued to elude her. This affected all other areas of her physical movement.

We had established a website for helping other disabled and disadvantaged children and their parents who were also searching for answers and solutions. Through this website, **www.littlestangel.com**, we had that moment of "awakening" for which every parent of a disabled child searches. Denise and I came across information that would change Rebecca's life and propel her development. It proved, beyond a doubt, that "life is stranger than fiction."

To our amazement, our further investigation and research showed that "unsubstantiated alternative medicine" for children with cerebral palsy was based on much more substantial basic science and medical research than were the accepted mainstream medical treatments.

For a year, we studied recent discoveries of brain injuries regarding the "penumbra" of the injury loci. We discovered that this penumbra of injured and/or metabolically inactive cells could make a substantial difference in a child's development.

This concept was not entirely new to me. Twenty years earlier, as an undergraduate in the University of Vermont's Medical School, Department of Neurobiology, I had conducted research on the central nervous system nerve regeneration. At that time, researchers had simplistically viewed nerve regeneration as something lower vertebrates could accomplish, but higher vertebrates could not. That is where all the research interest remained (as far as I knew). I was not aware that some researchers had discovered that there was a factor like a "penumbra" to assist in helping brain-injured patients.

The idea of a penumbra of brain cells really excited us because it gave us something that was possibly recoverable to work with. Up until that time, we had based our therapies on the concept of "neuronal plasticity"; that is, a neuron's ability to sprout new connections to effect movement learning.

The next questions we had to answer: "How to best proceed?... and where to go for treatments?"

After much research and thought, we had almost settled on trying hyperbaric treatments (HBOT) rather than vasodialator drug treatments for several basic reasons. But we were, oh, so tentative about taking the first step. Every physician and neurologist we spoke with about the idea told us that these techniques were "not proven." More important to us, they said that HBOT treatments would provide nothing to Rebecca...and could make her worse. The gamble of injuring Rebecca was too much for us to even consider.

Then, once again, fate interceded. While attending an education class in Chicago, my wife and I met two mothers who spoke highly of the specific motor skill gains their children had achieved with hyperbaric treatments. One of the mothers suggested we go to Canada for treatments because it was less expensive. The other mother told us to go to a "Dr. Neubauer" in Florida because he was the most experienced.

We immediately left Chicago and returned to our home in California. From there, Daddy, Mommy, and Rebecca flew on to Florida to meet "Dr. Neubauer."

Prior to starting the HBOT, Dr. Neubauer recommended we take a SPECT scan to determine the current condition of Rebecca's brain. The SPECT scan session was quite painless and without incident. Because Rebecca had to lie still for about one-half hour, she was given a small dose of valium to quiet her down. Despite that, she was an active five year old, and she wanted to look around. She was, however, her usual cooperative self. When I requested that she continue to lie still, she did so.

When I first saw her SPECT scan results, I cried. The extent of her brain damage was clearly obvious. I kissed Rebecca a hundred times that day in appreciation of how well she responded in spite of this extensive damage. After 36 HBOT sessions, I saw her next SPECT scan. Again, I cried. This time I cried because her response to HBOT was very obvious and equally extensive. I kissed Rebecca a hundred times that day as well. I knew we were on the right path to helping her reach   her potential.

When we arrived at the Ocean Hyperbaric Center in Lauderdale-by-the Sea, Florida, I spoke to Dr. Neubauer briefly about the conference that he was planning to hold...and then Rebecca and her Daddy entered the hyperbaric chamber for the first time.

This was a big afternoon! I felt an exhilaration and excitement over the prospect of what *might* come to pass. For the first time since Rebecca's birth, there was real hope that we were about to see the beginning of new progress and an end to a part of her past therapies. Rebecca had been told that she was getting a new therapy, and like the good soldier she is at all times, she did just what was required of her.

As we became pressurized, Rebecca became very active. At first, I thought it was from the excitement of being in a very small space with Daddy — what fun! But as time went on, I determined that it was more than just excitement; it was because of her response to HBOT. It "woke" her physically and gave her an energy level that was not unique, but is often attained as a result of HBOT. From the first, there was obviously something going on with her physiologically that seemed very positive.

After only six sessions, we took the weekend off to visit Rebecca's Florida grandparents for the weekend. I had noticed that her movements had more control and were much more smooth when she moved or reached for something.

More importantly, we also discovered, quite by accident, that for the first time in her life, Rebecca could swallow "thin" liquids without choking. The only reason we tried the orange juice without "thick-it" added was because we had forgotten to pack it in our travel bags.

Swallowing liquid without an additive was a major step for Rebecca, as swallowing is a very complex movement requiring many muscles to work in harmony. Before her HBO treatments, Rebecca could only drink highly "thickened" liquids; these liquids had to be made to a gelatinous consistency. Even then, she would still choke from time to time. What a wonderful surprise to discover her ability to drink regular drinks. All of us were elated.

It soon became apparent that Rebecca had made more significant advances in the first six sessions of HBOT than she had in four years of speech therapy and two and one-half years of feeding therapy! From that moment on, Rebecca, her mommy, and her daddy have been fully convinced of HBOT's immediate and long-term benefits.

Even though most chambers are basically alike, it is how the craftsman uses the tool, and not the tool itself, that is the mark of a great artist.

As a parent with a child with severe cerebral palsy, my strong advice to parents who are considering HBOT for their child is this: Go to the absolutely best center you can get to regardless of cost or travel issues. It is so important that you choose a center that will set you off on your journey on the right path, with the right compass and an accurate map. This is why we traveled from California to Florida to the Ocean Hyperbaric Center. We had learned through our research that it was the best and most experienced center in the U.S., if not the world.

Since that time, Dr. Neubauer has introduced us to other centers so that our travel burden would be lessened. But it was our experience and training in safety at Ocean Hyperbaric Center that gave us the knowledge to be able to discern some important safety features and quality differences that helped us in our search to locate an appropriate center that is geographically closer. First, however, this center must comply with Rebecca's needs, treatment nuances, and safety considerations. Because we started out correctly, we feel we can make such decisions with confidence as we move forward.

Today our current dilemma is how to integrate Rebecca's HBOT with her other weekly movement therapies. We think that will give her better development, with less work and effort. As I've said in other places, the need to keep finding the best system for a special child requires ongoing research, time, and effort.

The second thing that is critical in selecting a center is how they measure progress. It is essential to know where you are starting from and to be able to measure progress with some accuracy through a viable methodology. Dr. Neubauer has aggressively pursed imaging technologies to help his patients make decisions about whether HBOT is helping a child or not. The use of SPECT scans clearly documented for us where Rebecca's brain was active and where it was inactive. Taken again after appropriate treatments, we were able to see where changes were taking place. Consequently, my second advice to parents is that the find an HBOT center that uses SPECT or PET scans to determine the efficacy of the HBOT treatments.

Now, with our knowledge of HBOT safety and Dr. Neubauer's clinical experience, combined with the information we have gleaned from the various SPECT scans, and the way Rebecca has responded to HBOT, we feel we are in a good position to go to a different HBOT center with minimal risk.

After her first dose of hyperbaric oxygenation treatments, Rebecca went to see her wonderful neurologist, Dr. Asaikar, for her semi-annual check-up. We had not told Dr. Asaikar about our decision to have Rebecca undergo hyperbaric oxygen treatments...and we did not tell him where she had been at the beginning of the check up.

Dr. Asaiker could not stop praising Rebecca's progress. He was absolutely amazed at the progress she had made in six months. He was equally amazed at the changes in her brain scans.

Two months later, Rebecca's therapists unanimously noted that Rebecca had passed her plateau, gained more control, and had better tone and flexibility.

She was progressing faster than she had ever done before!

After Rebecca's second set of hyperbaric oxygen treatments, we focused on her physical therapies, primarily on movement therapy in hopes of "programming" newly awakened neurons. Soon we saw substantial changes and greatly improved head control.

Halfway through her third set of treatments, Rebecca began speaking. It was only a few words, including "good" and "yogurt," but we were thrilled. We had waited for so long to hear her speak. She was thrilled as well. It was obvious to us that she knew what she was saying as we asked her questions that could be answered only by those words.

In our delight, we ran up a sizable phone bill as we called all of our family to tell them of this wonderful advancement. Then, about three weeks after we returned home to California from one of our periodic trips to Florida, another miracle happened. As I do each night, I kissed Rebecca good night and said, "I love you." Only this time was different. She looked right back at me with her smiling eyes and said, "I love you." To me...for the very first time! We cried together in joy.

Every injured child is unique. Each one differs in his/her innate abilities, home life, and family. They also have a personalized response to their brain injuries and treatments. Therefore, each child's journey is formulated exclusively and while in motion.

A misstep here, and a successful shortcut there. And, while the final destination is relatively unknown, the child will most assuredly arrive at a far better destination than is otherwise possible or even hoped for if given the proper chance to overcome their impairments.

We know that one of the special ways our daughter was helped was through hyperbaric oxygen treatments. We will tell other parents, as we were told, that they should check it out.

We are now fully convinced that once the injured neurons have been re-established through HBOT, we must teach these unprogrammed neurons what to do and usefully integrate them into the nervous system.

For this reason, at the same time, we have continued to investigate, and sometimes incorporate, different therapy modalities and equipment into Rebecca's care plan.

How will history judge us? By how we have touched the lives of others.

Rebecca, in her very short, feeble, and challenged life (so far), will have greater stature and more memories than we could ever dream of. Not that she, herself, has accomplished so much, but that she has done so much after being given so little. Throughout her challenges and problems, she awakens each morning with a smile on her face, and struggles with Olympian determination at every therapy session. Every day she reminds us that her only purpose on this earth is to help others.

In time, history will view with favor the dedicated physicians and humanitarians, like Dr. Neubauer and his peers, for their lifelong and dedicated work conducted amidst controversy and disbelief. But, as a parent, I like to think they will be remembered not only for their great genius, but will also be remembered because they worked so hard to help a little girl whose heart and love are so great.

Rebecca is a new girl! We are now halfway through her projected 200 hyperbaric treatments. Her SPECT scan demonstrates that her brain is metabolically active throughout. We are now going for "depth," re-awakening of her penumbra neurons in the deeper parts of her brain. We are searching for the best way to integrate the remaining HBOT with movement therapies.

Our journey is certainly not complete, but I know that we are on the right path. I feel confident that we will reach our goal that Rebecca will have a very full, active, and independent life.

We now live a life of hope, expectation, excitement, and direction. Gone is our despair, broken spirit, and wondering about what to do to help her achieve her potential.

"Whom should I believe, and what should I do?" This is the most often spoken dilemma of parents of CP and brain-injured children. Inasmuch as very few physicians agree on how to "manage" these children, no wonder parents are confused. Even fewer physicians are in agreement on whether to "treat" the injury itself. The only "treatment" at this time is HBOT; all other therapies focus on treating the symptoms to "manage" the problem.

The truth is, treating neurologically injured patients is still very much in the dark ages of medicine. With all of the tremendous discoveries and advancements mankind has made in medicine, and in studying the human brain, we still have far more questions than answers.

As I've previously said, we have been exceptionally blessed with finding some of the most dedicated pediatric neurologists and physical therapists. In every case, they have worked wonderfully with Rebecca. Yet for many of her medical issues, we have had more questions and debates and conflicting answers from these exceptional practitioners than we've had answers. This has included defining and treating her seizures, deciding on the proper therapies, and, of course, whether or not to pursue HBOT.

We first saw an HBOT testimonial article in a popular South African magazine. But on the advice of medical professionals, we delayed pursing HBOT for two years. Then, as we heard more about HBOT, we did serious medical research for another year prior to starting HBOT treatments. Today, I wish I had understood HBOT when Rebecca was born.

What should a parent do? This is my advice to parents: Research your child's condition as quickly as possible. Among other things, investigate HBOT. Talk to a doctor who has had direct experience with it; don't take the advice of a doctor who has only read about it. Then find the most experienced HBOT center to begin treatments. Talk to other parents and learn how their child has reacted to HBOT. Know your own child.

As Denise has often said, "No therapist, physician, neurologist, or other trained, dedicated person knows your child like you do." Only her mommy, Rebecca, and I fully understand just what she needs. We will live the rest of her life with her challenges so we need to be actively involved in her medical care.

If we were to begin our journey again, from that fateful day, September 10, 1995, when Rebecca chose to live, our very first step would be into a hyperbaric chamber for treatments. This would have enabled us to most assuredly attain our destination more quickly and more directly...and much less painfully.

In closing this story, let me say that we will continue to give Rebecca hyperbaric oxygen treatments in a chamber for as long as she continues to show improvement.

We also send our best wishes to all the "friends of Rebecca," and send them our prayers while they struggle on their journey to reach their potential destination.

Rebecca, Ed, and Denise Nemeth
April 29, 2001

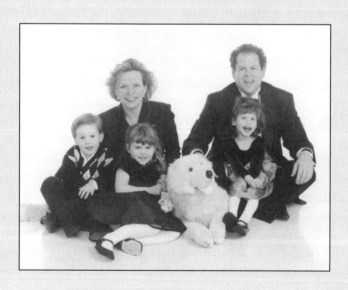

HYPERBARIC CHAMBERS: THE DELIVERY SYSTEM

Hyperbaric chambers, when properly installed and well maintained, provide a safe treatment facility for hyperbaric medicine.

—Dan McNeil, President
PVHO$_2$ Systems, Inc.

Introduction

Until the early 1960s, most hyperbaric chambers in the United States were operated by the military, especially the Navy and the Air Force. They were used primarily to support programs for diving- and altitude-related work and experiments. By the late 1970s, one of the primary users of hyperbaric chambers was the commercial diving community, and in the early 1980s, recreational diving groups began using hyperbaric chambers with great frequency as well. During this period, decompression sickness accounted for most of the treatments performed in hyperbaric chambers. Today, it is estimated that the use of hyperbaric chambers for diving incidents represents less than 3% of all hyperbaric medical applications. The tremendous and astonishing growth of the use of hyperbaric chambers for medical purposes in the 1990s occurred because of the progress made in understanding the extent of medical problems caused or exacerbated by hypoxia (lack of oxygen).

Today, the evolution of the use of hyperbaric oxygen therapy in military programs, commercial and recreational diving communities, and ultimately in the medical field, continues to move at a rapid pace. The acceptance of hyperbaric oxygen therapy is becoming more extensive in the U.S. This has resulted in a proliferation of different types of hyperbaric chambers. As with any type of medical equipment, however, not all brands or all types of hyperbaric chambers are suitable for every type of treatment. Therefore, when discussing the value of hyperbaric oxygen therapy, it is always important to realize that treatment will be only as effective as the quality and type of equipment used to supply oxygen under additional pressure.

The piece of medical equipment required for administering oxygen under hyperbaric conditions is commonly referred to as a hyperbaric "chamber," although most hyperbaric chambers more closely resemble large, enclosed capsules with windows. There are some chambers, mostly in other countries, that are the size of a very large building; these facilities often have several rooms. When evaluating various hyperbaric centers, it should be noted that many types of chambers, found in different types of medical facilities, are not necessarily the best ones to use for HBO treatments for children with cerebral palsy or traumatic brain injuries.

Types of Chambers

Hyperbaric chambers are usually classified according to the number of people who can use the chamber at one time. Class A chambers can hold two or more people and are secured in a fixed location. They are usually referred to as multiplace or "walk-in" chambers. Class A chambers have the capacity to lock people in and out under pressure and usually require extensive support and control systems. In some of the large chambers in Canada, there is room for 11 - 12 children, each with a parent.

The Class B chamber is a single occupancy chamber; this is usually referred to as a monoplace chamber. For many years, Class B chambers were constructed as small, moveable cylinders made of clear acrylic for maximum visibility. In recent years, Class B chamber designs have become more sophisticated. Some small chambers now have auxiliary personnel chambers to allow for patient care, and other manufacturers are producing monoplace chambers with acrylic tubes that are much larger in diameter than the early models. A few manufacturers are producing chambers that use compressed air rather than oxygen; in these chambers, the patient is given oxygen by a mask or hood.

Class C chambers are used for testing purposes. These chambers are designed for animal occupancy only.

Chamber classifications in the United States are issued by the National Fire Protection Association (NFPA-99 Health Care Facilities). Furthermore, all chambers used for clinical applications in the U.S. must be designed, fabricated, and installed in accord with the American Society of Mechanical Engineers (ASME)-Pressure Vessels for Human Occupancy (PVHO-1). This helps to ensure that welding processes, procedures, and materials are in accordance with established standards. This agency also enumerates the qualifications necessary to work with specific chambers, and ensures that the acrylic windows in the chambers are constructed in accordance with ASME/PVHO-1 standards.

Different models of multiplace (Class A-multiple) and monoplace (Class B-single) chambers are used in many countries for treating children with cerebral palsy and traumatic brain injuries. In the United States, however, the chamber most commonly used for the treatment of cerebral palsy and brain injuries is the monoplace chamber, because there is no technician needed in the chamber and the patients can be treated at individual protocols. Although there are some excellent centers worldwide that use multiplace chambers, there is some debate concerning the appropriateness of using multiplace chambers in the treatment of children with cerebral palsy and/or brain injuries.

There are advantages and disadvantages to using either monoplace or multiplace chambers.

Monoplace Chambers

At this time, most monoplace chambers are cylinders made of metal or acrylic with metal ends. They are usually designed so the patient can lie horizontally or recline in a semi-sitting position. These are the most widely used types of chambers in the U.S., as they allow for more flexibility and individual monitoring and care. In most centers, monoplace chambers are designed so that they cannot be pressurized above three atmospheres absolute (ATA). This provides added protection to the patient. Because of horizontal positioning, the patient can be transferred into the chamber from a gurney if necessary. The acrylic sides allow full visibility of the patient by the supporting hyperbaric technician.

There is also a model that allows the patient to sit up, watch television, listen to music, or lie back and rest. Some monoplace chambers are designed to have enough room to allow a caregiver to accompany a child into the chamber.

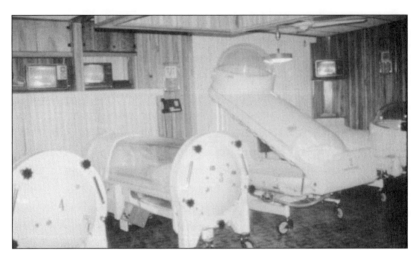

FIGURE 1 Various designs of monoplace chambers

All chambers are required to have built-in communication systems so the patient can speak to the technician. Monoplace chambers use one of two types of oxygen flow mechanism. The first type is constant purging. An adjustable rate of oxygen flows through the chamber and out again to the external environment.

As discussed previously, monoplace chambers are currently the most commonly used for children with cerebral palsy and traumatic brain injuries. The advantages of the monoplace chamber are as follows:

1. The patient is allowed privacy, and the chance of secondary infection is reduced.
2. There is no need to wear a face mask or hood (this is important with children).
3. In most cases, it is more comfortable than a multiplace chamber, and there is no chance of an ill-fitting mask or hood allowing oxygen leakage.
4. If the patient is confined to a gurney, it makes for an easier transfer into and out of the chamber. For patients who are unable to move about by themselves, the monoplace chamber is much more convenient for the technicians who work with them.
5. It is easier to observe each patient as an individual. (With children, it allows both the caregiver and the hyperbaric attendant to observe

the patient without disturbing anyone else.) This is also an advantage for children who are restless, spastic, or who involuntarily cry out.

6. The monoplace chamber can be moved to different locations and/or in and out of a facility for cleaning or repair. Additionally, it can easily be turned to the correct angle of the television set; this makes it easier for different sized people to watch television and/or be supervised by the hyperbaric technician. In the usual configuration, one hyperbaric attendant can sit between two chambers and observe both occupants.

7. Infants can be treated in a monoplace 100% oxygen chamber as they do not require hood drivers or masks.

Like any other type of pneumatic machinery, there are also some minor disadvantages. Working with experienced operators and properly maintained equipment can greatly reduce any difficulties that might be encountered:

1. Oxygen supports combustion. Hyperbaric centers must have stringent safety procedures, and attendants must be well trained and experienced due to the fire hazard associated with using pure oxygen. To be specific: the pressure of oxygen is increased when pressurized in a chamber. [100% of oxygen = 100% x (ATAs − 1) = PO_2. Example: 100% oxygen x (3 ATA −1 = 2ATA)= 200% PO_2.]

2. Communication with the patient is most often by way of a microphone. This microphone can be plugged into the individual chamber on an "as needed" basis whenever the patient needs to speak to the hyperbaric technician or vice versa. Some models have communication centers built in. As with all equipment, the more that is added to the chamber, the more expensive it becomes, and the more there is to maintain to ensure complete safety to the patient.

3. Due to limited space, hospitals and rehabilitation centers with large numbers of patients needing physical therapy cannot carry out therapy inside a monoplace chamber.

Portable Monoplace Chambers

There are several types of monoplace chambers that are transportable for use in the diving field, where expert medical help is several hours away from working commercial divers or underwater construction workers (i.e., working on a deep tunnel). There are also chambers specifically designed to be used in high-altitude work or climbing. These chambers are designed to be used in emergencies until the injured diver can be transported to a free-standing, multiplace hyperbaric chamber or a chamber incorporated into a hospital or other specialized medical facility.

In addition, monoplace chambers made out of a very substantial fabric are becoming more available. While they may in the future play a role in treating children with cerebral palsy and brain injuries, scientific research must still be conducted to determine the safety and effectiveness of these chambers.

Multiplace Chambers

A multiplace chamber usually has a capacity of two to five people, but some multiplace chambers can accommodate up to thirty-six persons. These patients can all be treated at the same time. In the multiplace chamber, the entire chamber is filled with pressurized air. Pressurized oxygen breathed by the patients is delivered by a mask or a hood that covers the head. In a few multiplace chambers, each patient can be given oxygen at an individualized percentage; in most chambers, however, all patients are given the same percentage of pressurized oxygen for the same amount of time.

Manufacturers of hyperbaric chambers bring out new models periodically, often with minor changes. Changes might be made to improve procedures, patient comfort level, or aesthetic aspects of the chamber. For example, some of the most modern multiplace chambers are air-conditioned to control humidity and temperature.

In some countries (i.e., Japan and Russia), multiplace hyperbaric chambers are frequently used as operating rooms for surgical procedures. Although a special type of chamber is required, major procedures such as open heart surgery can be performed. In China, chambers are frequently used for cardiac surgery without the necessity for heart and lung by-pass procedures used in typical heart surgeries of this type.

The advantages of the multiplace chamber include the following:

1. A large number of patients can be treated simultaneously.
2. There is a reduced fire hazard as the chamber is filled with air.

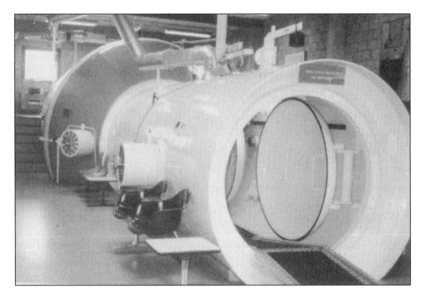

FIGURE 2 A multiplace chamber

3. For special circumstances, such as decompression sickness or air embolism, the pressure can be increased above 3 ATA.
4. When appropriate, physical therapy and surgery can be conducted in the chamber.

Other types of mobile multiplace hyperbaric chambers have primarily special uses such as sports physiology, physical therapy research, treatment of patients with cerebrovascular insufficiency, myocardial ischemia, and peripheral vascular disease. They are also used for conducting mental exercise experiments and for emergency treatments when several patients are too far away from standard facilities. It is not uncommon for professional football and hockey teams to have their own chambers for safe and timely treatment of injured players or for players who need to recover quickly from exhaustion.

Hyperbaric Chamber Maintenance

Hyperbaric chambers are very durable pieces of equipment; this also makes them quite expensive. A well-made monoplace hyperbaric chamber purchased new will cost approximately $100,000; a multiplace chamber will cost from $250,000 to $1 million plus. For the most part, it is not the age of the hyperbaric chamber that is critical, but the daily care and ongoing maintenance that are consequential to the health and safety of the patient. As stated earlier, most chambers in the U.S. are constructed according to the specifications of ASME codes as established by ANSI-ASME/PVHO (American National Standard Institute). Chambers built to these codes, or similar codes from other countries, have the structural integrity to give many, many years of reliable service when properly maintained. Therefore, when selecting an HBOT center, it is important to question not only the type of hyperbaric chamber that will be used, but also the system used for maintaining it.

It is the responsibility of the manufacturer to establish receiving, in-process, final inspection, and testing activities when new equipment is installed. After that, there must be proper procedures established for the maintenance schedule to ensure that periodic calibration, testing of pressure in the chamber, and inspection of all hardware take place. This type of periodic inspection and maintenance requires the services of an experienced hyperbaric chamber technician.

Chamber Operations

The essential controls of the average monoplace chamber are on the exterior of the hyperbaric chamber where they can be continually monitored by a trained hyperbaric support technician who monitors the gauges and operates valves or regulators. The most basic pressure control systems use manually operated valves to adjust the chamber pressure. The technician has the responsibility of observing the occupant of the chamber as the pressure gradually increases. Once the chamber has reached the treatment pressure, the hyperbaric technician monitors the chamber pressure gauge to ensure that the pressure remains constant during the treatment phase. Technically, treatment time starts when the pressure inside the chamber reaches the level prescribed by the attending hyperbaric physician. It is very rare that the patient ever encounters any problems while in the chamber, but the safety-conscious center will operate only when there is a board-certified hyperbaric physician in charge.

As with all forms of equipment and/or machinery, the exact location of the controls will not be the same with all manufacturers. These control gauges are similar in the different brands of quality hyperbaric chambers, although the placement and names of the controls may differ. For safety reasons, there is no electrical power inside a chamber. In the monoplace chamber, the opening and shutting is done with a hand crank or locking door cam for added safety.

Safety in the Chamber

When all precautions are taken, the incidence of fires in chambers is quite small. For example, in 75 years of using chambers, there have been less than 120 fatalities, worldwide. To realize how small that number actually is, one has only to compare it with the 90 deaths that occur each year in sport diving in the United States. (Over the course of 75 years, this would amount to a total of more than 6,000 fatalities.) Because there is the chance of fire unless strict safety standards are enforced, conscientious chamber centers are extremely careful.

Fires are caused by a combination of factors rather than a single problem. Three factors must be present for a fire to take place: ignition, fuel, and oxygen. The source of ignition is commonly static electricity generated by improper clothing worn by patients, although ignition can occur as the result of any kind of electrical spark (i.e., created by faulty equipment or friction). In addition, a fire must be supported by some form of fuel. Any flammable materials present in the chamber can act as fuel—clothing, paper, etc. Oxygen is the final component that must be present for a fire to take place. Fire cannot be maintained in the absence of oxygen. Furthermore, the intensity of a fire is determined by oxygen concentrations. In short, higher oxygen concentrations result in more intense fires.

Thus, adherence to safety guidelines and maintenance standards is imperative in ensuring proper chamber function and safe delivery of treatment. Fire prevention is the most important component of any safety program related to hyperbaric chambers. There are increasingly stringent regulations to ensure compliance with all applicable standards and manufacturing requirements involved with the design, fabrication, and installation of hyperbaric chambers. It is critical that caregivers determine that a hyperbaric center not only have, but also strictly enforce, its fire-prevention standards. When these standards are upheld, chances of fire are greatly reduced. Thorough investigation has found that all instances of fire or explosion are due to human error, carelessness, and/or lack of attention to prescribed safety precautions.

Fire is a greater hazard in a monoplace chamber than in the multiplace chamber because the monoplace chamber is filled with pure oxygen. To prevent any chance of fire or explosion, the following instructions for patients undergoing hyperbaric oxygen therapy apply to any monoplace chamber pressurized with pure oxygen:

1. Only 100% cotton clothing and undergarments should ever be worn inside the chamber. It is important to avoid wearing all synthetics, nylons, or other similar fabrics. Cotton is the only fabric known to never cause static electricity. Children who wear diapers can keep them on, but they should be as clean and dry as possible before entering the chamber.
2. Watches, wigs, hairpins, any kind of jewelry, prosthetic devices, hearing aids, contact lens, or any substance or object that may cause a spark must be removed before entering the chamber.
3. No one should undergo hyperbaric oxygen therapy when there is any grease or oil on the skin and hair. This means that all suntan lotion, perfumes, hair sprays, nail polish, facial creams, body oil, and makeup should be carefully removed before undergoing the HBO therapy.

The caregiver must be alert to anything that might injure a child, and should work with the hyperbaric center technicians to be certain that all safety precautions are strictly followed.

There are additional precautions that should be observed as well:

1. The only foreign object that should be taken into the chamber is unwrapped hard candy or a piece of gum without wrapping. Even unwrapped hard candy or gum should be approved by the hyperbaric technician before it is taken into the chamber. Of course, any kind of hard candy or gum should be given only to patients who are old enough and physically fit to suck or chew without danger of choking.
2. The technician should be advised if the patient has had ear infections or may have trouble clearing the ears.
3. Patients who are diabetic should eat something before a treatment, but like all other patients, they should avoid gas-producing foods or drinks to avoid gastric discomfort.

4. Patients should continue to take routine medications, including insulin, prior to the treatment.

5. All seizures or high temperatures that occur prior to or between hyperbaric treatments should be reported before entering the chamber.

6. It is best if the bladder is empty before taking treatments in a hyperbaric chamber because the increased pressure makes all cavities of the body have a tendency to compress slightly.

Problems in the Chamber

It is rare that a patient experiences any pain while undergoing HBO treatments. Occasionally, a patient will experience some ear discomfort. The spaces in the ear containing air that are of concern in hyperbaric medicine are the two middle ear spaces and the paranasal sinuses. Pain in these areas is commonly referred to as a "squeeze." It is caused by the difficulty (sometimes inability) of the patient to equalize pressure in the middle ears or sinuses during compression or decompression. Most people can minimize the chance of this pain by frequently yawning, swallowing, or blowing the nose with the nostrils pinched and the mouth closed; these techniques are known as modified Valsalva maneuvers, and are usually the most effective in pressure equalization. On very rare occasions, children who are too young to understand this instruction will need to have a tube inserted in their ears. Some centers in the United States require a child to have a ventilation tube before hyperbaric oxygen treatments.

Conclusion

While the general appearance of hyperbaric chambers has not seen extensive revision through time, their purpose and function continue to evolve. From multiplace chambers constructed to accommodate more than a dozen people to monoplace chambers built to hold a single patient, technological advancements allow for improved efficiency, safety, and comfort. A variety of organizations have established strict regulations to help ensure the safety of patients receiving hyperbaric oxygen therapy, and their stipulations for construction, maintenance, and periodic inspection of hyperbaric equipment can assist caregivers in selecting an appropriate and well-managed facility for the treatment of their children.

SELECTING AN APPROPRIATE HBOT CENTER

Introduction

In the United States, there are approximately 500 - 700 hyperbaric centers that treat a variety of illnesses. Only a small number of these chambers are used for the care of children with cerebral palsy or brain injuries. Many chambers are used exclusively for treating diving accidents; some chambers are used for training new commercial divers through simulated dives. Hyperbaric chambers may be located in hospitals, medical centers, or commercial diving schools, and a lesser number are free-standing units. Most hyperbaric centers are used primarily for wound healing and accidents involving a sudden loss of oxygen to the body due to carbon monoxide poisoning, smoke inhalation, or serious burns caused by fire or radiation. Some centers treat several types of diseases such as multiple sclerosis, Lyme disease, and reflex sympathetic dystrophy in addition to strokes and traumatic accidents, and some centers offer a combination of these services.

The most critical aspects of evaluating a hyperbaric center are not the combination of illnesses and accidents the center treats, or the location of the center. Rather, the staff, equipment, safety features, and appropriate protocols are factors that should be considered.

Important Considerations

Hyperbaric medical treatments should be the primary service of a free-standing center; HBOT should not be an adjunct to another business unless the hyperbaric center or department is part of a large medical complex or educational institution. Currently, there are a number of excellent centers in various parts of the United States and Canada that have the skilled staff, equipment, and experience to treat children with cerebral palsy or brain injuries.

Caregivers should be aware that there are centers advertising treatment for children whose services are not satisfactory. Some of these centers are not staffed with adequately trained medical personnel; others do not have the right types of equipment. A few have less than acceptable safety standards, and many are not equipped to determine which part of the brain has been damaged, or to document the value of hyperbaric oxygen therapy.

Caregivers must thoroughly investigate the HBOT center they intend to use for treatment. Not many private physicians have sufficient background in hyperbaric oxygen therapy or knowledge of the various centers to be able to guide the caregiver. It is imperative that the caregiver ask questions on the phone or request the center to provide evidence of its expertise and experience. When the initial visit takes place, the caregiver should make certain that all questions and concerns are fully addressed. It is sometimes prudent not to schedule a treatment on the first visit; this will make it easier to decide for or against using a specific facility. Ask for the cost of the treatments in writing to avoid unfortunate surprises at the end of the therapy.

Most importantly, be certain that the staff has medical training, proper protocols, and experience with this treatment modality. You are the one responsible for the health and welfare of the child. Therefore, you have both the right and the responsibility to make certain that the therapy is safe and effective.

Staff Qualifications

The individual in charge of a medically sound hyperbaric facility should be an experienced physician with a degree from an accredited medical school. He or she should have experience working with hyperbaric oxygen therapy and preferably have board certification. If in doubt, ask to see the doctor's degrees and certificates, and inquire where he or she received specialized hyperbaric oxygen therapy training. It is also important that the physician have experience working with children who have cerebral palsy or other types of brain injuries. Medications and oxygen pressures must be adjusted in relationship to any improvements shown by the child during the course of HBO treatments. The physician in charge must know at what level the oxygen therapy should be given, as this can change on a frequent basis. For example, even though caregivers are frequently told that exposure to a pressure of 1.5 - 1.7 ATA for a period of 45 minutes to 2 hours is the safest and most effective treatment for a child with cerebral palsy, these levels must be decreased to 1.1 to 1.5 for children with cerebral palsy who suffer from seizures. Inasmuch as 50% of all children with cerebral palsy suffer from some type of seizure, this is a critical point.

The rest of the staff is equally important. Individuals most likely to be qualified to work with children who have cerebral palsy or brain injuries will be experienced nurses, paramedics, technicians, and, perhaps, a doctor who is completing an internship in hyperbaric medicine. In addition to their basic training and experience working with children, the staff administering the treatments must have a thorough knowledge of the use of oxygen under increased pressure and specialized training in the proper operation of a hyperbaric chamber. If the center you are considering doesn't supply you with this type of information in writing or during your initial consultation, be sure to ask for proof of expertise.

Facility and Equipment Safety

It is also critical that you know what type of HBOT equipment the facility uses and the safety procedures it has installed to ensure that the equipment and oxygen therapy are safe. Pure oxygen is a highly flammable gas. It has the potential for both explosion and fire if not properly handled. Inasmuch as even a spark of static electricity can cause an explosion, it is entirely proper to inquire how the facility enforces safety standards.

Although there are several types of chambers that are effective to use for HBOT, there is definitely a right and wrong way to set up and maintain them. While you may not have expertise in hyperbaric chambers, you will want the center you are investigating to explain how the chambers are operated, and especially how they are maintained. You may also want an explanation of how the pressurized oxygen is administered and the precautions that are taken.

Evaluation Procedures

If an HBOT center does not have a SPECT scanner, it should have a comparable system for use before and after HBO treatments. The system needs to clearly document that the brain has areas that may be revitalized by oxygen under increased pressure. Furthermore, the center should be able to scientifically demonstrate that the therapy is helping the brain to function more effectively. The caregiver should have the reassurance that HBOT is a viable treatment for the child, and that there is a reasonable possibility that some of the child's physical and/or mental deficiencies will decrease. Like any other treatment modality, not all children are helped by HBOT in the same way. In some cases, HBOT does not seem to have any effect on a child's condition. The actual documented rate of successful improvement is approximately 85%.

Experience with Hyperbaric Oxygen Therapy

It may be helpful in evaluating a center to inquire how long the facility has been in operation as well as the name of the owner or medical doctor. Length of time is not the most essential factor, but if the center has been in operation only a short time, it may mean that the staff has less experience in administering treatments. If the center is new, it is appropriate to ask where the hyperbaric doctor and staff received their training in this field. The length of time that a center has been in operation is not as critical as the past experience and training of its personnel.

It is also prudent to ask to review any written or published materials the center has prepared. Most established hyperbaric centers will be happy to send you a packet including information that answers many of your questions.

If you are in doubt about the physician, you may want to read some of the papers that he or she has published on the subject of hyperbaric oxygen treatment for children with cerebral palsy or brain injuries. You may also consider asking for a list of conferences he or she has attended and/or a list of presentations given at these conferences. At this time, many of the most experienced hyperbaric physicians are actively taking part in studies, writing papers, and making presentations at medical conferences in an effort to document new ideas and procedures.

Conclusion

For caregivers who are unfamiliar with hyperbaric oxygen therapy as a treatment option for children with cerebral palsy or brain injuries, it is essential to learn as much as possible in order to make an informed decision about the most effective course of action to take in a child's care.

Understanding the procedures and safety measures that a facility employs is of the utmost importance in choosing a HBOT center. Ask questions, request information, and make a preliminary visit to ensure that all safety measures are being met and the staff is fully qualified to treat the child in your care. The child's safety is always a priority, and a quality treatment facility will respond to your concerns and make every effort to demonstrate its competency.

THE POSITION OF THE MEDICAL COMMUNITY AND INSURANCE COMPANIES

*HBO is a drug delivery system that makes the vital drug
oxygen available to the injured brain tissue. Its physiologic
and pharmacologic applications cannot be duplicated by
any known drug or combination of drugs.*
—Sheldon F. Gottlieb, Ph.D.

Introduction

As discussed briefly in other chapters of this book, hyperbaric oxygen therapy is a medical treatment accepted by the American Medical Association (AMA) and approved for payment by Medicare for 14 different medical conditions. At this time, however, HBOT has not been universally approved for use with children who have cerebral palsy, nor do many medical facilities use it for children with brain injuries. Until HBOT has been formally approved by the AMA and is prescribed by the majority of the U.S. medical community for children with cerebral palsy, insurance companies will be reluctant to pay for treatments beyond the scope of the 14 conditions that have already been approved.

Doctors and HBOT

For a variety of reasons, the majority of medical professionals, including pediatric neurologists and most pediatricians, do not as yet fully understand or agree with the benefits of hyperbaric oxygen therapy for children with cerebral palsy or traumatic brain injuries. First of all, most doctors are not familiar with hyperbaric medicine because it is not a part of the standard curriculum in medical schools. Doctors must spend their own time and money to seek additional training in the specialized field of hyperbarics.

In addition, many practicing physicians rely on the advice of the Food and Drug Administration (FDA) to formally approve a drug or medication before using it. The purpose of the FDA is to protect citizens from drugs that may be more harmful than beneficial. This special protection has functioned as a safeguard for the consumer many times in the past. But to gain FDA approval is a very expensive and lengthy process. It is estimated that the cost of securing FDA approval of a drug or procedure through tests and studies is approximately $250,000 - $500,000, and can take from two to five years. Inasmuch as oxygen is not a new "drug," this process is not required by the FDA. Approval is left to be decided by other organizations such as the AMA and Medicare.

Many conscientious and excellent physicians are extremely cautious about recommending new treatments for children with cerebral palsy. This is to be admired, as there are many new treatments, procedures, and types of equipment that may not meet their manufacturers' promotional claims. A doctor's hesitation is in the best interest of the patient, especially when he or she knows little about the treatment in question, or when confronted with the decision of whether or not to prescribe a treatment that is controversial. Yet while this hesitation is meant to protect the patient, it may also hinder the improvement of his or her condition. Physicians may advise caregivers of children with cerebral palsy to be cautious and wait for controlled, double-blind studies to prove the effectiveness of HBOT. Unfortunately, such studies are not forthcoming.

There are two primary reasons why there are no controlled studies to date: cost and ethical considerations. Such studies cost between $250,000 and $1 million. These studies are usually financed by pharmaceutical companies, but a profit-oriented company will only fund studies that will prove the value of a new drug they are interested in marketing. In addition, it is very difficult to ask the caregiver of a child with cerebral palsy to participate in a study in which only half of the children involved will receive any benefit. Some researchers believe that this is an unethical way to treat any patient who must already cope with a multitude of health problems.

Alternative Testing Methods

Most medical professionals who say that more research is needed, or that they are waiting for the results of controlled, double-blind studies, do not thoroughly understand the difficulties involved in applying this test to hyperbaric oxygen therapy. (Keep in mind that the principal behind a double-blind study is that neither the patients nor the doctors have knowledge of which patients are receiving the active treatment.) When a patient undergoes HBOT, he or she is immediately aware of pressure changes in the chamber. In a double-blind study, patients would know whether or not they were receiving pressurized oxygen, which would thus render the study invalid. Furthermore, such a study is impractical because it would be impossible for the physician to monitor the condition of his or her patients or to make recommendations for changes in treatment.

When a child with cerebral palsy receives hyperbaric oxygen treatments, the caregiver often makes note of increased flexibility, decline in seizures, and overall improvement in the child's condition. While this in itself does not qualify as a controlled study, the observations of caregivers and physicians, as well as use of the SPECT scan as a method of measuring brain function, serve as forms of positive verification of the effectiveness of HBOT. A child may also act as "his or her own control," meaning that when a child begins hyperbaric oxygen therapy and no other aspect of the child's treatment regimen has been altered, any changes in the child's condition are caused by the introduction of the new therapy. This is another method of verifying the effectiveness of HBOT for children with cerebral palsy.

Continuing Education

Many experienced, practicing physicians receive updated information on medical protocols and current research from literature provided to them by pharmaceutical companies. Additionally, these companies offer a variety of courses and workshops to doctors who wish to earn continuing education credits to keep their medical licenses current, or who simply have a desire to acquire more information on particular topics. However, because pharmaceutical companies do not consider oxygen to be a drug of importance, they neither distribute information on the subject nor design courses for doctors who have an interest in hyperbaric medicine. Oxygen, under pressure, is considered to be a drug by the FDA. However, oxygen is a free commodity found in air and available to everyone.

To cultivate a better understanding of hyperbaric medicine within the medical community, and to share information on the latest clinical studies, research, and procedures, an international symposium on various new treatments for children with cerebral palsy took place in the summer of 2001. This symposium was attended by physicians, caregivers, researchers, and other proponents of hyperbaric oxygen therapy for children with cerebral palsy. Speakers from ten different countries presented information on the progress of this treatment. The symposium also offered continuing education credits, which gives an indication of the growing positive interest in HBOT.

Conclusion

The path to obtaining understanding and approval of a new medical therapy is not without obstacles. It requires time to demonstrate its safety and usefulness to the medical community. There is a definite need for controlled, double-blind studies for new medications and therapies, but this type of study need not be the only method of proving the effectiveness of a treatment. The thousands of children who are showing significant improvement in spasticity, vision, motor control, and cognitive abilities should be adequate proof for physicians to begin investigating and learning more about this type of therapy. If the average physician fully understood the theory behind the use of HBOT for children with cerebral palsy and traumatic brain injuries, and saw the results of clinical studies, there would be greater support for this form of treatment.

A BRIEF SUMMARY OF WORLDWIDE RESEARCH, CLINICAL STUDIES, AND OTHER USES OF HYPERBARIC OXYGEN THERAPY FOR CHILDREN WITH CEREBRAL PALSY AND BRAIN INJURIES

Enlightenment cannot enter the closed mind.
—W.I. Neubauer (1977)

Introduction

This chapter provides a brief introduction to information published in medical journals, presentations at hyperbaric conferences, and discussions among the growing number of hyperbaric physicians and researchers concerning the use of HBOT in cases of children with chronic brain injuries. The studies and reports listed here also cover a wide range of topics related to hyperbaric oxygen therapy including both formal and informal clinical studies. This review is generally limited, however, to studies that have been or are currently being conducted related to cerebral palsy and brain injuries. While the studies presented in the following pages are only a fraction of the hundreds of those being conducted around the world, they represent the diversity of countries that are now taking an interest in HBOT as a viable treatment option in cases involving children. These studies have been instrumental in verifying the importance of HBO as a component of the therapy regimen for children with cerebral palsy.

Controversy Regarding HBOT

In a report issued in 1999 by the American Academy for Cerebral Palsy and Developmental Medicine, United Cerebral Palsy Association (USA), available on their 2001 website (listed as "Status Report on Unsubstantiated Interventions"), the following statement explains the association's position on the subject of hyperbaric oxygen therapy:

> The clinical usefulness of hyperbaric oxygen therapy in the treatment of disabilities associated with cerebral palsy is presently based only on individual anecdotes. Its usefulness has not been put to the test using research methods essential for its evaluation.
>
> A few clinical studies have been reported; a few pilot studies utilizing organized protocols of evaluation are said to have been done, but the methodologies and their results have not been published in the peer reviewed scientific literature.
>
> Although not yet demonstrated, it is conceivable that hyperbaric oxygenation may be of help to selected persons with certain kinds of disabilities. If it is helpful, it is not known whether beneficial effects are short-lived or permanent. It is also conceivable that any positive results at best are marginal and/or temporary. Finally, it is conceivable that hyperbaric oxygenation has no beneficial results.

While this statement seems to cast hyperbaric oxygen therapy in a negative light, it actually leaves room for additional research and keeps open the possibility of officially recognizing HBOT as a treatment for children with cerebral palsy.

Furthermore, the 2001 webpages of the United Cerebral Palsy Association (USA) include this statement:

> During the past few years, a few clinicians have explored the use of hyperbaric oxygenation in a variety of conditions such as stroke, head injury, spinal cord injuries, and multiple sclerosis. At this time, the published scientific literature does not support the use of this technique in any of these conditions. A major problem has been the lack of well-designed clinical trials utilizing a scientifically acceptable protocol to evaluate the usefulness of the procedure for these conditions. There is no scientifically acceptable evidence at this time that demonstrates its [HBOT's] clinical usefulness; neither

is there any scientifically acceptable evidence available at this time demonstrating its lack of usefulness. Individual stories ("anecdotes") tell very little; they are interesting, provocative, but not scientifically informative.

Again, this statement allows for the possibility that HBOT might be approved after further testing, specifically tests meeting the parameters required for a controlled, double-blind study.

Definition of Terms

The definitions provided below will aid the reader in understanding the conditions that are established when a study is being conducted.

Control Group

A control group is composed of subjects closely resembling the treatment group in many demographic variables but not receiving the active medication or treatment under study. These individuals thereby serve as a comparison group when treatment results are evaluated.

Controlled, Double-blind Study

A controlled, double-blind study is one in which neither the doctors nor the patients know which patients are assigned to the control group and which are receiving the active treatment. Individuals in the control group are given an inert substance known as a placebo.

Pilot Study

A pilot study is a preliminary or experimental trial or test that does not necessarily meet the same requirements as a controlled, double-blind study.

Crossover Study

This type of study makes conditions more equal for both groups. First a patient receives either a medication or treatment for one half of the study and none for the second half of the study. The other group does the opposite; they begin the study with the placebo and receive the actual treatment during the second half of the study. Of course, neither knows when or what they are receiving.

Delayed Entry Trial

Participants are assigned to start the trial at different times, but are usually matched as to age, size, medical problems, and severity of the problem. For example, one group begins the study six months after the first group and thereby serves as a control.

A Brief Review of Important Studies

The majority of studies listed below were presented at the 2nd International Symposium on Hyperbaric Oxygenation in Cerebral Palsy and the Brain Injured Child in July 2001. The actual papers on the various studies included in this chapter are contained in *Proceedings of the Second International Symposium on Hyperbaric Oxygenation in Cerebral Palsy and the Brain Injured Child*. For convenience, these studies on HBO are listed in alphabetical order. This publication is available through your local bookstore or Best Publishing Company.

Brazil

One of the physicians to make the earliest reports on the use of HBO for children with cerebral palsy was Dr. J.J. Machado. In 1989, at the New Horizons in Hyperbaric Medicine Conference, Dr. Machado reported on the reduction of spasticity for children with cerebral palsy when using hyperbaric oxygen therapy. At that time, Dr. Machado was making observations of patients he had been treating since 1979. He stated, "from that time [1979], we have used it [HBOT] as an adjunct to physiotherapy in the rehabilitation of these patients." This was one of the first times that a physician had publicly informed others in the medical field of the use of hyperbaric oxygen therapy for children and adults with cerebral palsy.

At a conference that took place in 1999, Dr. Solany Zerbini presented results of a follow-up study of 232 patients from a group of more than 2,000 patients, aged 1 - 34, that she and her associates had treated during a 25-year period. She provided the following statistics [as reported by the patients]: 40% improved in spasticity, 40% in attention, 10% in memory, and 13% in comprehension. At the 2001 conference, Dr. Zerbini reported on an update of her studies and stated that patients continued to confirm approximately the same statistical results.

Bulgaria

A report from Bulgaria entitled "The Effects of Hyperbaric Oxygenation on Psycho-Motor Functions by Children with Cerebral Palsy" was presented by Ivan Chavdarov, M.D., Ph.D. He is associated with a specialized hospital for residential treatment of prolonged therapy and rehabilitation of children with cerebral palsy. In his report, he states that "Since 1997 till now we have used hyperbaric oxygenation as an important part of the management of children with cerebral palsy and we combine it with other therapy methods."

Canada

Some of the most publicized studies on the use of HBOT for children with cerebral palsy have been conducted in Canada, with the most recent (and, perhaps, the most controversial) study taking place in 2000. Led by Dr. Jean Paul Collet under the auspices of McGill University, the purpose of the study was to determine if the use of HBOT could result in improvement in gross motor function. One hundred and eleven children participated in the study, with 57 being randomly allocated to the treatment group and 54 being randomly assigned to the placebo group (also known as the control group). All children received 40 treatments over a period of two months. The treatment group received 100% oxygen at 1.75 ATA while the placebo group was exposed to ambient air (21% oxygen) at 1.3 ATA. It was established from the onset that this was to be controlled, double-blind study.

Two important points must be kept in mind: 1) a placebo is defined as an inert substance having no effect on the body, and 2) neither the patients nor the physicians are aware of which individuals are receiving the active treatment in a double-blind study. In order for the study to be valid, researchers determined that the placebo group would receive ambient air at a slightly elevated pressure, such as would produce a "masking" effect and a change in chamber pressure that would be perceptible to the patients.

The results of the study were startling. By the end of the treatments, both groups demonstrated improvement in gross motor control. Even more surprising was the fact that both groups experienced the same degree of improvement. Despite these positive results, the findings of the study were reported in a negative light. Rather than conclude that the "placebo"—a lower concentration of oxygen delivered at low pressure—could be just as effective as higher concentrations of oxygen at higher pressures, it was reported that hyperbaric oxygen therapy was found to have no greater effect on patients than an innocuous placebo and that no further research in this area should be conducted. However, it must be noted that his study was serendipitous, in that the more severe cases reacted more effectively and more quickly with the 1.75 ATA hyperbaric treatments than did the severely affected control patients. In addition, what was termed an innocuous placebo was in fact not totally inert. Dr. Philip James states in the *Lancet* (June of 2001) that "compressed air at 1.3 ATA increases the plasma oxygen tension from 12.7 kPa (95 mm Hg) to 19.7 kPa (148 mm Hg), and to increase the concentration of such a reactive substrate by 50% is certainly notable." Therefore, this was not a true placebo. This study reopens the area of compressed air therapy dating back to the 1930s and the outstanding work of Orville Cunningham (See page 129). Debate concerning the validity of this study is far from over.

China

There are more than 1,800 hyperbaric clinics in China, and it is estimated that 10,000 physicians, technicians, nurses, and research scientists are trained to treat the nearly 90,000 patients who seek treatment for a multitude of problems each year. At the 11th International Congress on Hyperbaric Medicine, held in Fuzhou, China, Dr. W. Qibiao presented a paper on his successful treatment of children with epilepsy using HBO, demonstrating effectiveness in 82% of the children with significant effectiveness in 68%.

Drs. Lianbi Xue and Hai Yu, et al., of the Department of Hyperbaric Oxygenation, Naval General Hospital, Beijing, are currently studying the effects of hyperbaric oxygen on brain bFGF and bFGF mRMA expression on neonatal rats after hypoxia-ischemia injury to discover if this mechanism may be related to clinical usefulness of HBO for cerebral palsy. At the same time, Dr. Xue is conducting an ongoing study of the effects of hyperbaric oxygenation on children with brain injuries. His initial report indicates that the results of HBO are satisfactory, invariable, and permanent.

Cuba

Dr. R. Castelianso and Dr. C. Galvez are conducting studies on the pediatric indicators of hyperbaric oxygenation use.

Germany

H. Wassmann, M.D. of the Institute for Neurophysiology in Munster, Germany, along with a group of associates, is conducting studies to investigate the use of HBO in cases of cerebral palsy. Their findings indicate that there is a distinct benefit from HBO therapy, especially in younger patients. The focus of their study is on cerebral energy crisis in vitro and in vivo under hyperbaric oxygenation.

Japan

During the 13th International Congress on Hyperbaric Medicine in Kobe, Japan (1999), several interesting papers were presented on the use of hyperbaric oxygen with various types of injuries. Drs. Chen Jianhui and Lin Shaohua presented their findings that the effects of HBO in the treatment of brain stem injury are remarkable. "HBO is able to increase consciousness, shorten the course of the illness, and increase the rate of cure. Specifically, the treatment group had a cure rate of 68% and a death rate of 5.6% while the other group had a cure rate of 36% and a death rate of 40%."

Mexico

In the 1960s, a group of physicians in Mexico City began to take newborn infants with severe cases of hypoxia (lack of oxygen) from the delivery room into the hyperbaric chamber as a standard practice. It was reported that there was a lower frequency of disabilities, and children who did experience effects of hypoxia required fewer treatments to prevent potential damage. This practice was discontinued in the 1970s, but Dr. E.C. Sanchez and his colleagues are currently proposing that a study be conducted to demonstrate that neonates can be adequately treated in a monoplace chamber to prevent cerebral palsy.

Russia

The portion of the former USSR that is now Russia has more than 3,000 chambers. The exact number of chambers in other parts of the former USSR is not known, but it is estimated that they also have several thousands. HBO has been used for many years in the early stages of cerebral palsy and is also frequently used to treat serious brain injuries.

Dr. N.V. Kazantsea published a paper in which he reported that a new method of using increased oxygen pressure in the chamber may be effective. Dr. Kazantsea and his associates experimented with reduced pressures to determine their effect on cerebral palsy and other neurological injuries. They named this method of manipulating oxygen pressure Minimized Hyperbaric Treatment (MHT).

A paper by Dr. M.A. Labov entitled "Hyperbaric Oxygenation in the Treatment of Cerebral Palsy in Childhood" reports that during the course of his study, some of his patients experienced a dramatic improvement and prompt regression of motor deficiencies, but the method was ineffective for other children. Dr. Labov found that the best results were seen in children less than one year old and those with spastic hemiplegia and diplegia.

Sicily / Italy

A medical team of father and daughter, B. and A. Sparacia, are doing a great deal of research on the effects of hyperbaric oxygenation. This includes studies of children in the womb and investigations of free radicals. In a paper published in EUBS in 2000, they presented their study on the compounds which are now widely recognized to play a key role in the pathogenesis of tissue damage in various organs and systems.

In another study, A. Sparacia reports on the value of using HBO for mothers involved in high-risk pregnancies. She has found that giving HBO treatments to expectant mothers with medical complications can often decrease the risk to the fetus. In her study, Dr. Sparacia and her associates found that HBOT is irreplaceable in improving both placental blood flow and oxygen diffusion at the cellular level. Furthermore, this study hypothesized that "if the metabolic effects of hyperbaric oxygen on cell enzymes and hemocoagulants are taken into account, the multimodal action by hyperbaric oxygen is undoubtedly important in starting the delicate treatment of fetal growth defects and, more generally, of pregnancies at risk."

Other uses of HBOT studied by the Sparacias have included cerebral blood flow determination in ischemic brain damage, treatment deficiencies in fetal growth, and the rationale of HBO in preeclampsia therapy. Dr. B. Sparacia, the senior doctor, has been involved in this field since the early 1990s.

South Africa

There are several centers for treating patients with HBO in parts of South Africa. Some of these centers are similar to the centers of the UK hyperbaric trust program. Although there have been few published articles of the work conducted in this country, it has been reported that the positive results are compelling. Dr. F.J. Cronje and his associates have released a position paper, "The Use of HBOT in the Treatment of Children with Cerebral Palsy," which concludes that more scientific studies are needed before such reports can be verified.

United Kingdom

In 1963, J. Hutchinson, et al. published an article in the *Lancet* on the use of hyperbaric oxygenation in severely cyanotic children. These children were exposed to extremely high pressure (4 ATA) for brief periods. Although this level of pressure is now considered excessive and inappropriate in the treatment of infants, the statistical percentage of recovery for these children was positive.

The United Kingdom now has 110 chambers operating as a center known as the Hyperbaric Oxygen Trust. Under the direction of Dr. Philip James, the center is dedicated to the use of HBOT for children with cerebral palsy and brain injuries. A study of the children who have been treated at the Hyperbaric Oxygen Trust supports the belief that HBO is an effective therapy in cases of children with cerebral palsy. Dr. James is currently writing a book including a chapter entitled Suffer the Little Children on his postive findings in CP and the brain-injured child. Although his book has been designed primarily for physicians and professionals in hyperbaric medicine, explanations of scientific data also make the book accessible to the lay person.

United States

Despite the fact that research concerning HBOT in the United States has lagged behind work being conducted in other countries, innovative physicians and scientists have been working the field of hyperbaric medicine since the early 1970s. As early as 1972, the American Journal of Surgery published articles related to oxygen supply in healing wounds. This is the same concept that Dr. Edgar End adopted in developing the theory that brain tissue would react to HBO in much the same way as the other tissues of the body.

Physicians and researchers in the field of hyperbaric medicine have recognized the necessity of sharing information through publishing their work and presenting their research at symposiums and conferences. Reports on the effects of hyperbaric oxygen therapy for children with spastic diplegic cerebral palsy were published in the *Undersea and Hyperbaric Medicine Journal* in 1999 and presented at the 1st International Symposium on Cerebral Palsy and the Brain Injured Child, held in Boca Raton, Florida in 1999 and the 2nd International Symposium held in 2001.

One of the more recent studies on children with cerebral palsy was conducted by Dr. Maurine Packard of Cornell Medical Center in 2000. It was designed as a randomized, delayed entry trial of the effects of HBOT on a small group of children, aged one to five, with moderate to severe cerebral palsy. Over the short trial period, all children were exposed to oxygen at increased pressure at various times, some beginning immediately after enrollment and the others within six months. The results of the study were as follows: "For some children with moderate to severe CP, there is evidence that HBOT improves motor skills, attention, language, play, and...for some, an increase in vision..." Furthermore, "The main differences between HBOT and traditional therapies are the rapid gains over brief periods of time and the impact on cognitive skills..." It was noted that some regression occurred mainly in motor tone, with a return of spasticity which may well be related to the protocol and may not have included the necessary number of treatments in each case. Dr. Packard concluded that "Further blinded studies are needed to discern whether some of these effects are secondary to prolonged parental interactions."

Conclusion

As can be noted by the diversity and number of studies currently being conducted, HBO is being demonstrated to be successful specifically for moderate to severe cases of cerebral palsy. Contrary to the position currently outlined by the leading cerebral palsy organizations, there is increasing evidence that HBOT can assist children with cerebral palsy to improve their motor skills, attention, language skills, and, in some cases, their vision.

When a caregiver and/or the child's physician or therapists see a change in the child's skills and behavior after HBO treatments, it must be considered that the HBO treatments have contributed to the cause of these improvements. However, to satisfy the medical profession and to validate without question the value of hyperbaric oxygen therapy for children, further research is needed. Controlled, double-blind studies will be required to objectively substantiate that the effects of HBOT are realistic and long standing.

ADDITIONAL TREATMENTS FOR THE CHILD WITH CEREBRAL PALSY OR A TRAUMATIC BRAIN INJURY

*Although there is no one therapy approach universally recognized,
neuro-development is enhanced by physical, occupational, and speech
therapies based on dynamic and changing neuro-anatomical principles...
these therapies play an undeniable role in functional
outcomes for children with brain damage.*
—Raymond H. Cralle,
Registered Physical Therapist

Introduction

The primary focus of this book is on the positive benefits often achieved when a child with cerebral palsy or a traumatic brain injury is given an appropriate and timely dose of hyperbaric oxygen therapy. It is fully recognized, however, that HBOT is only one form of therapy a child usually needs. In most cases, hyperbaric oxygen therapy is given as a complementary form of therapy. In nearly all instances, the child continues with physical, occupational, or speech therapies and appropriate medications even while HBOT is being administered.

This chapter contains only a brief introduction to a wide variety of more traditional therapy modalities which are often used to provide assistance in motor control, walking, and general improvement of the quality of life for children with cerebral palsy. The chapter also briefly introduces some of the supporting types of equipment and medical techniques used with these children. Like HBOT, the goal of therapy and/or supporting devices, techniques, and equipment is to help each child function at his or her maximum capacity.

The inclusion of the different forms of therapy is intended to give a caregiver a broad idea of the wide range of therapies, medications, and equipment currently being used as well as a few systems which were once widely used but are not often used today. Because not all systems work for each child in the same way, it is the role of the therapist and the pediatrician to help caregivers determine which therapy, or therapies, best meets the needs of a specific child. As noted above, HBO is not intended to replace the other therapies recommended by the child's physician and healthcare team, but rather to complement them.

For convenience, information is divided into three sections: Types of Therapy, Supportive Medical Interventions, and Equipment and Devices. Topics within these sections are introduced in alphabetical order to prevent caregivers from forming the impression that they are listed by value or preference. They are NOT listed in order or popularity, frequency of use, or recognition by the medical profession and/or cerebral palsy organizations. Caregivers searching for assistance in deciding which form of therapy or what equipment is best to use may find it somewhat discouraging that this chapter does not give them this specific type of information. The reader must understand that it would be unrealistic and irresponsible to discuss the pros and cons of the different therapies and treatments without knowing the individual child. Each child is unique and the necessary type of therapy or equipment will depend on the severity of the child's condition. Other characteristics that must be taken into consideration include the age of the child, the personality and attitude of the child toward the specific therapy, the attitude of the caregiver, the caregiver's level of involvement, and the ability of the caregiver to finance the various forms of therapy, equipment, or transportation costs. Also to be considered are the length of time that has passed since the brain injury occurred and whether the caregiver is also giving HBOT to the child. Therefore, it is hoped that the list of therapies and support equipment presented below will increase caregivers' awareness of the treatment options that are available to them, and will encourage further research based on the needs of individual children and their families.

Equally important, however, is a word of caution. Just as there are many high-quality therapists who are well trained in physics, physiology, psychology, and various forms of therapy, there are some individuals who call themselves therapists who do not have adequate qualifications. Caregivers are cautioned to thoroughly investigate any type of therapy or system of alternative or complementary medicine. The same caution applies to any equipment used, devices purchased, surgeries recommended, or promises which seem "too good to be true." At the same time, caregivers must recognize that their local pediatrician may not be well versed about new types of therapy. Sometimes the best places to gather information are on the Internet, through parent groups, or referrals from other parents. Often it takes a combination of factors and quite a bit of time for a caregiver to know which therapy will be most beneficial to the child's special needs.

Selecting a Competent Therapist

Most qualified therapists are highly educated and specialists in their field. They not only incorporate a number of types of therapy in their work, but also are receptive to new and creative therapy methods. New clinical information is being uncovered continually, and competent therapists are constantly applying this new information to their work. Awareness of new ideas, an understanding of different types of therapy, and an open mind to possible new techniques are indications of a therapist who is seeking what is best for the child.

Specialists Who Assist Children with Cerebral Palsy

Specialists who work as a team must also develop effective and ongoing communication patterns with the other members of the support team as well as the caregivers to facilitate the best service for the child. While each specialist is concerned with his or her special therapy treatment, the idea of a global approach best serves the overall needs of the child. In addition to medical personnel, the three primary types of therapists a child with cerebral palsy or a traumatic brain injury usually has on a healthcare team are the occupational therapist, the physical therapist, and the speech therapist.

Occupational Therapy

The main function of an occupational therapist who specializes in working with children with cerebral palsy is to develop the functional tasks which require small motor skills. This type of therapy is especially important for children who have problems with their upper extremities. An occupational therapist will usually develop a treatment pattern that supports the natural maturation process and tries to discourage abnormal motor behavior.

Depending on the type of cerebral palsy or the degree of severity, the therapist may help the child develop the skills needed to operate a computerized keyboard or to write legibly. For other children, the goal may be to improve functions involved in the tasks of daily living, or to determine the best positions for optimum stretching and/or exercising the hands. This is especially important for a child who is wheelchair-dependent. Although rare, the therapist may also be involved in helping a self-abusive child by giving the caregivers methods for protection and prevention. Some occupational therapists make hand splints; others are specialists in seating recommendations.

Physical Therapy

Physical therapists and occupational therapists have a tendency to overlap in their work with children with cerebral palsy because both therapies involve helping the child develop motor skills. The physical therapist, however, is primarily concerned with large motor activities that involve the legs; this includes working with the muscles necessary for walking, bracing, using crutches, and/or rehabilitation after surgery. One major difference between the occupational therapist and the physical therapist is that the occupational therapist is involved in having the child complete activities that will assist growth through motivation. The physical therapist, on the other hand, works directly on the child's body to help alleviate muscle tightness or lack of tone, and usually develops a plan for continuation of the work when the child is at home.

Nutritionist

Sometimes a child will experience little weight gain as an infant, or there will be a weight loss because of poor nutrition. If the physician feels that the child is not getting the proper nutrition because of oral motor dysfunction, the problem will usually be referred to a speech therapist. In other cases, the weight loss may be due to the types of food the child prefers or is willing to chew. The role of the nutritionist is to help the caregiver develop a menu of foods that the child can and will eat that also provide the nutrients the child needs.

Speech Therapy

Many children with cerebral palsy have problems with their oral motor system. Some do not speak at all; others have difficulty speaking properly and/or eating and swallowing. A speech therapist is usually needed to diagnose and treat these problems.

A speech therapist may specialize in evaluating the process of eating, teaching phonation, or a combination of both. The speech therapist, who is involved in the feeding process, must first evaluate the mechanical process of eating which involves several movements to properly handle food. The therapist needs to know how the food is moved in the mouth to the back of the throat, how effective the swallowing mechanism is, and in what position the child can handle mouth muscles most efficiently. Gathering this information often requires a comprehensive examination using different textures of food. In many cases, it also involves special x-rays to observe the swallowing mechanism. Based on the evaluation, the therapist will make recommendations about where to place the food in the mouth, how thick it should be, the need for special textures, and suggestions for feeding the child in a specific position to avoid choking. The speech therapist (or another specialized therapist) will next evaluate the child for speech skills. The medical term for people who have difficulty with speech, especially coordinating and articulating words, is dysarthria; this condition is most common with children with athetosis. The focus for children with dysarthria will be on teaching them how to breathe and use the vocal cords to make sounds.

Eating, swallowing, and speaking are areas that have a tendency to change as the child matures; further evaluation as the child grows may be necessary. The speech therapist is often involved when a child has a problem with drooling (sialorrhea). Drooling treatment involves a care team approach with the coordination of a dentist, ear, nose, and throat physicians, the pediatrician, and seating specialists. The primary role of the speech therapist is to teach the child to make every attempt to keep the mouth closed and to swallow the saliva.

Types of Therapy

The better known forms of therapy, developed before 1980, are the Phelps, Deaver, Brunnstrom, Fay-Doman, PNF, Bobaths, and Rood methods. Each of these therapies uses one or more of the following systems: stimulus, labyrinthine reflexes, tonic neck reflexes, righting reflexes, postural reflexes, synergic patterns, orientation, strength, range of motion, ontogenetic patterns, phylogentic patterns, and/or bracing. The majority of physical and occupational therapists use an eclectic approach, selecting from the various treatment systems, approaches, and latest scientific data. Many other forms of therapy have also been developed since that time, but they generally continue to incorporate aspects of the systems listed above.

Biofeedback Modification

Many behaviors exhibited by a child with cerebral palsy, such as head-banging, self-injuries, and/or severe spasticity, can be helped through the use of biofeedback devices if the child is cooperative and the caregiver strictly follows the behavior modification program. Biofeedback is based on the theory that if the child is given feedback about an unwanted position or behavior, and is rewarded each time for correcting it, the child will learn to use the more acceptable behavior or postion.

Bobaths

(See Neurodevelopment Therapy)

Brunnstrom

Brunnstrom used synergistic muscle patterns in his treatment system. He also developed a system of treatment for adult hemiplegics that used an offshoot of this system to help individuals gain control over the predictable flexor and extensor synergies so that multiple combinations of these movement patterns could be used.

Equine Therapy

In this type of therapy, also called hippotherapy, the child is placed on horseback to learn balance and relaxation. It is theorized that the rhythm of the horse's movements causes the muscles to relax so that it is easier for the therapist to work with specific groups.

Fay and Doman

(See Patterning)

Kabot and Knott Theory

This therapy is based on the idea of using the whole limb and/or multiple joints rather than focusing on individual joints and muscle groups. The principle behind this therapy is that the movements that are the most useful are those involving an entire part of the body rather than isolated muscles. This is a combination of the theories of Kabot and Knott. Kabot originally developed techniques to overcome muscle weakness from paralysis. Knott extended Kabot's methods and applied them to other forms of neuromuscular deficiencies.

Myofascial Release Therapy

Myofascial release is one of the relatively new additions to the types of therapy that are being used in physical therapy today. It is somewhat different from traditional therapies in that it is generally an extremely mild and gentle form of stretch. Although it may appear to the patient that not much progress is being made during a treatment, the end result is often a profound increase in mobility and lack of tightness in the body's tissues. As idicated by the name, the process attempts to gradually release the fascia from its tight constraints that are holding parts of the body stiff or in pain. Inasmuch as one of the two forms of fascia covers nearly every part of the body, when it hardens or loses its elasticity, it becomes difficult to move portions of the body. This therapy was originally an outgrowth of chiropractic techniques and is based on chemical theories plus stretching and manipulation. The overall goal is to stretch the connective tissues involved in joint capsules and in the fascia overlying the muscles to reduce pain and to allow the patient to move freely.

Neurodevelopment Therapy (NDT)

NDT, developed by Bobaths, is based on the concept that children with cerebral palsy often need assistance moving through various stages of development. This theory espouses the belief that it is important for children to go through these phases in the appropriate order to accomplish proper development. In this therapy form, children are encouraged to roll over before they sit, and to crawl before they try to walk.

Patterning

Developed by Fay and Doman-Delachtro, this therapy is based on the concept that human movement evolves from immature to sophisticated movements. Therefore, the patient begins with simple movements and progresses toward more sophisticated movements to ingrain the movements in the brain. This therapy, at its most demanding, has the family organize teams of helpers who work with the child for hours each day repeating the same motion over and over so that the brain will learn and retain it.

Phelps Theory

This theory focuses on the use of braces and working on the active and passive range of motions, and is based on the theories used with polio patients.

The Portage System

The Portage system is designed to be a home educational program. It consists of 580 skills that the child learns in sequence. In this case, the parents are the therapists.

Rolfing

This therapy method involves deep massage, followed by stretching and manipulation. It is thought that this combination can help the muscles relax and have less spasticity. For the most part, this very deep muscle therapy is quite strenuous to the patient's body both during the therapy and for several days afterward.

The Rood Method

Margaret Rood introduced this system of therapy that uses heat, cold, bushing, and other similar methods to eliminate stimuli that are thought to make certain areas of the body initiate specific movements. Treatment attempts to overcome this abnormal stimulation by desensitizing those affected areas that cause the foot to grip, etc. This system focuses attention on the gamma motor system and stimulation of the nervous system, particularly through exteroceptors.

Sensory Integration

First introduced by Jean Ayres, sensory integration is designed to help children with decreased sensory input execute movements more effectively. The theory behind this therapy is that many children with cerebral palsy have difficulty with movement because their sensory motor neurons are impaired. Sensory integration involves a large amount of activity, passive touching, and movement stimulation. It is intended to help the brain initiate more appropriate movement patterns. For many of the exercises, the therapy incorporates swivel chairs and hands-on exercises.

Trigger Zone Therapy

The goal of this therapy is to find trigger points that cause positive reflexive actions and stimulate them so that the action is imprinted on the brain.

Supportive Medical Interventions

Alcohol and Phenol Injections

A popular technique for treating cerebral palsy for many years involved injecting alcohol or phenol into the nerves or muscles to weaken or paralyze very spastic muscles. These injections were often quite painful and needed to be done under anesthetic. It was discovered, however, that both alcohol and phenol damage the nerves and muscles and delay normal functions, so they are rarely used today. (See BOTOX)

Amino Acid Therapy

Amino Acid Disorder is a genetic defect that prevents the body from converting one amino acid (phenylalanine) to another (tryosine). If left untreated, it results in mental retardation, seizures, and imperfect hair pigmentation. It is possible that some prenatal damage occurs to the brain of a child with this disorder, but the earlier in life that treatment begins, the lower the incidence of seizures. After proper treatment, the electroencephalograph tends to return to near normal. Early treatment includes a diet low in phenylalanine.

BOTOX Injections

BOTOX (botulinum toxin) can be injected into muscles to weaken spasticity. This drug is injected with such a small needle that it causes very little pain and does not cause scarring. The effects last from four to six months, and it can be used quite a few times. BOTOX has been tested extensively, is approved by the FDA, and is often used for children who have only one or two involved muscles. It is thought to occasionally belay but not prevent development. For children with spasticity who are unable to undergo other types of therapy, BOTOX injections are sometimes the best way to control the problem.

Surgery

There are approximately 12 different types of surgery used to help children with cerebral palsy. The specific surgery is dependent on the level of involvement and the reason the surgery is needed. Some are quite successful for most children. Others are successful only about half of the time, and in some procedures, the surgery may need to be repeated as the child grows. The expertise of a neuropediatrician and/or a neurosurgeon is necessary to determine if a child needs surgery, and to estimate the potential success of a specific surgical procedure. Determining if and when to perform surgery to reduce spasticity or help a child walk requires a comprehensive individualized evaluation and the understanding of the caregivers that not all such surgery is fully successful.

Two surgical procedures that involve the brain and/or the spinal column are the dorsal rhizotomy which cuts the nerves coming from the spinal cord, and the less invasive surgery that involves placing a

114

pump under the skin of the abdomen. This procedure allows an anti-seizure medication to be added to the fluid surrounding the spinal cord.

The vagal nerve stimulator (VNS), also referred to as the "pacemaker of the brain," is a generator the size of a pocket watch that is implanted under the skin of the patient's chest. The lead wire from the device is then tunneled up the neck, and coils at the end of this wire are wrapped around the vagus nerve. Using a laptop computer and a programming wand, the neurologist programs the system to deliver regular mild electrical stimulation to the vagus nerve. Its use is directed mostly toward patients with intractable epilepsy. The system has been clinically proven to decrease, and, in some patients, completely eliminate, seizures in adults and children over twelve years of age.

Equipment and Devices

There are literally hundreds of types of equipment and special devices on the market today whose purpose is to help children stand more erect, walk more effectively, sit straighter, etc. Selecting the proper piece of equipment or device is another area where the caregiver needs to exercise caution.

Adeli Suit

The Adeli Suit is an adaptation of a Russian cosmonaut space suit designed to put the body in proper alignment and to provide feedback between the muscles and the brain. It is a form-fitting suit equipped with adjustable elastic bands. For children with cerebral palsy who lack motor control, the suit restricts the movement of the limbs. Patients go through rigorous physical therapy to help retrain the brain to understand the signals from correct muscle movements.

Braces

Although there appears to be no consensus among physicians about the benefits of braces, they are often used for back problems, feet imperfections, hips, ankles, and, at times, legs. The negative impact is that they tend to decrease functions instead of strengthen them. The positive effects are that they allow some children to perform tasks they would not otherwise be able to do.

Communication Devices

If the child is unable to speak because of spasticity of the vocal cords (or for other reasons), the speech therapist will evaluate the child to determine if the child is capable of using other means of communication. This would include hand signals, electronic computerized devices, symbol boards, or merely eye communication.

Gastrostomy

If the child aspirates or chokes on a regular basis, the specialized speech therapist may recommend a gastrostomy tube. There are two primary types of gastrostomy tubes. The first is the Stamm gastrostomy, which involves opening up the abdomen and placing a tube into the stomach. The second type, a percutaneous gastrostomy, involves inserting a needle through the abdomen into the stomach and sliding the gastrostomy tube over the needle during feeding times.

Quadriciser

The Quadriciser is a new advance in therapy equipment that has significant possibilities. This is a motor-driven system that moves cables and pulleys that are attached to the hand while gripping and cradling the foot. It has been called a major breakthrough in physical, psychological, and emotional therapy for the severely disabled child as well as the elderly. All four limbs are continuously moved and coordinated in a natural rhythm that simulates walking or crawling. The range of motion of each limb and the rate of movement may be customized with resistance so that high-symestic exercise occurs. Timed sessions and speed control provide a choice of duration and cardiovascular intensity.

Conclusion

For the caregiver, the decision to begin therapy leads to another important decision that must be made. There are many types of therapy to choose from, and hundreds of devices and types of equipment made to assist the child. It is impossible to thoroughly investigate each of these devices. For this reason, the caregiver often depends on the advice of the care-giving team to suggest what is most appropriate for a specific child's needs. The same is true of the type of therapy used. The role of the therapist, no matter how well educated or how experienced or what their specific expertise, is to assist the child in reaching his or her maximum potential.

THE HISTORY AND USES OF HYPERBARIC MEDICINE

There is nothing more difficult to carry out, nor more doubtful of success,
nor more dangerous to handle, than to initiate a new order of things.
—Machiavelli (1469 - 1527)

Introduction

The development of hyperbaric medicine and the evolution of hyperbaric chamber design are so entwined that it is nearly impossible to reflect on the development of the medical aspects without discussing the history of the chambers used to administer pressurized air or oxygen. Oftentimes, individuals who were medical pioneers of hyperbaric oxygen therapy also played a critical role in the development of the hyperbaric chamber. They were the inventors, designers, and manufacturers of the chambers they used for experiments and/or treating patients. In addition to their ideas about how the human body might benefit from the use of pressurized air, these individuals needed to understand complex mathematics and be proficient in engineering, construction, and the concepts of mechanical devices.

At times, there were overlapping discoveries about hyperbaric medicine in various parts of the world because scientists and medical professionals in the early years of hyperbaric medicine (the 1600s) were unable to share information due to limited means of communication. Furthermore, the era of widespread printing had not yet begun, so until the 1800s, they often had little if any written documentation about the work done by their predecessors or the construction of earlier chambers.

Thus, a scientist working on a new concept would neither have contact with others who were working on the same ideas in other parts of the world nor have access to anyone who had done previous work on the concept. For these reasons, the development of hyperbaric medicine sometimes had a lapse of 50 - 60 years between one major discovery and the next. Another reason for delays between advancements in hyperbaric medicine is that most individuals who were involved in this field completed their work without the support of their colleagues. The creative and innovative spirit demonstrated by doctors and scientists investigating hyperbaric oxygenation often led to their ostracism from the larger medical community.

Overall, the progress of hyperbaric medicine has been more sporadic for applications in the treatment of various medical problems than for use in the diving community. In contrast to the slow and often discouraging progress of hyperbaric medicine, the keen desire of man to go deeper under water kept the diving industry's interest in hyperbaric chambers high. Scientists, medical professionals, and manufacturers interested in diving procedures continued to move forward with their work. From World War I through the end of World War II, the military had the greatest interest in diving and the use of hyperbaric chambers. Later, when the world's attention became focused on the oil that lay deep in the oceans, diving companies spent millions of dollars to fund research in hyperbaric medicine in order to improve safety for commercial divers.

Whether utilized in commercial arenas or the medical community, hyperbaric oxygenation and the methods by which it is administered have changed dramatically through time. This chapter includes a brief overview of hyperbaric chambers, from the earliest historical accounts to current endeavors.

Diving and HBO

As mentioned above, the earliest development of hyperbaric medicine is connected specifically to the history of diving and diving medicine. For centuries, the human race has been fascinated by what is under the water. Records of breath-hold diving from 4500 BC indicate that divers were searching for mother-of-pearl. There are also written records from 400 BC of Xerxes using divers to repair his ships and to salvage goods from his enemies' sunken ships. According to these records, early divers were able to stay down for 2 - 4 minutes at depths of 20 - 30 feet.

One hundred years later, Alexander the Great was lowered in a glass barrel into the Bosphorus Straits.

The price paid by these underwater adventurers was various degrees of decompression sickness (the bends) and other complications, especially to their ears, lungs, and brains. It was the divers' desire to go even deeper, and the unpleasant physical consequences of these ventures, that eventually led to many of the applications that are now utilized by modern medicine in hyperbaric oxygen therapy.

Unsung Heroes

Progress and development in the field of hyperbaric medicine covers a period of nearly 350 years. From Xerxes and Alexander to today, all of these adventurers used the same theories of pressurization, but as time went on the systems that were developed for the production and use of pressurized oxygen became much more sophisticated.

There were hundreds of innovative physicians and scientists who contributed to the development of hyperbaric medicine. Their accomplishments, including pictures of the chambers they developed and built, are documented with drawings and photos in the book *History of Hyperbaric Chambers* by Gerhard Haux. This chapter has only enough space to cover the endeavors of a few of these individuals, but they each played an important role in the development of hyperbaric medicine as it is used today. The stories of their discoveries, their personal trials, and the animosity they frequently encountered in trying to gain the acceptance of the larger medical community make them true but unsung heroes.

These innovative men and women attempted to accomplish tasks that were not easy. Without electricity or modern manufacturing methods, the pressurization of the chambers and the methods they used to introduce a pressurized environment were very primitive by today's standards. Although their medical understanding and knowledge lacked sophistication, some of the early hyperbaric chambers that were designed and used had basic features that are still in use today, and their applications of hyperbaric oxygenation are currently being reevaluated.

The First 240 Years

During the first 240 years of research in hyperbaric medicine (1660 - 1920), progress was slow despite medical advances, developments in the field of engineering, and discoveries about medical uses of oxygen. The effects of oxygen on the body were not yet fully understood; neither was oxygen's potential for explosion if improperly handled. Several unfortunate incidents resulted from this lack of understanding, and the medical profession came to think that oxygen under pressure was toxic to the human body and far too dangerous to use. Despite these concerns, many physicians and scientists had a sufficient understanding of the body to continue their investigations about air and oxygen and their relationship with pressure.

1620

Around 1620, Cornelius Drebbel developed a one-atmospheric diving bell; this was basically the beginning of the idea of modern submarines. His purpose, however, was to help divers stay under water for longer periods of time.

1660

Robert Boyle, an Irish naturalist who was at one time the President of the Institutes of Science in London, joined forces with Gay-Lussac to develop the General Gas Law. This law states that the pressure of gases is inversely proportional to their volume at constant temperature. This law is still of utmost importance for any mathematical calculation related to HBO.

1662

An English clergyman named Henshaw built a pressure-tight chamber called a "domicilium." Its purpose was to improve the health of its users; thus, it was intended more for preventative treatment than for curing disease. Inasmuch as he used a pair of bellows to build up the inside pressure, it probably was not much above sea level, but he was certainly on the right track. Although he may not have had scientific evidence that he was correct, Henshaw said of his invention, "In times of good health this domicilium is proposed as a good expedient to help digestion, to promote insensible respiration, to facilitate breathing and expectoration, and consequently, of excellent use for the prevention of most afflictions of the lungs."

1774

Joseph Priestly, an English scientist, made the next known advancement in hyperbaric medicine when he discovered oxygen. He was responsible for the discovery of oxygen, as well as a variety of other substances including chlorine, ammonia, sulphurous acid, and carbon oxide. He also did work related to electricity and vision. Priestly used the newly discovered gas—oxygen (which he initially called "dephlogisticated air")—for wound healing. Until this time all chambers had used only pressurized air.

Priestly's theory of healing through oxygen therapy quickly met with disapproval when the French chemist Antoine Lavoisier (1743 - 1794) brought attention to the risk of oxygen toxicity. Lavoisier, a renowned scientist, was correct, and his report on the toxicity of concentrated oxygen on any organism was an important scientific discovery. However, his thesis on the danger of using oxygen for medicinal purposes did much to slow the development of hyperbaric medicine. Priestly resigned himself to the idea that "the air which nature has provided for us is as good as we deserve."

Despite the lack of acceptance of the use of pressurized oxygen for medical purposes, other scientists and physicians over the next 200 years continued to study its effects on the human body. It is important to remember that when these scientists were working on treating lung disorders and other diseases, many mechanical devices we take for granted had not yet been invented. For example, there were very limited ways to seal the doors that closed the chambers, and the idea of wearing masks or hoods to allow intake of oxygen had not yet been discovered. Furthermore, there was no general rationale for hyperbaric treatments. It is suspected that each physician merely prescribed treatments to his patients as he thought best.

1796

Beddoe and Watt wrote the first book about oxygen therapy.

1834

Junod built a chamber in France for the treatment of lung diseases and other pulmonary afflictions. Three years later, he constructed a larger chamber with a capacity of 12 patients. This was at the time the largest chamber ever built.

1836

Pravaz built Germany's first hyperbaric chamber. His was a stand-up chamber, as were most chambers up to this time. This creation became the largest chamber in the world. It was used to treat a wide variety of ailments. In his time, there was no way to measure or estimate the partial pressure of oxygen in the blood, so the results of his work are speculative.

1855

Eugene Bertin, a French medical doctor, wrote a book about his personal hyperbaric treatment center and its results; his book includes the first published drawing of a pressurized air chamber.

During this same time period (1850 - 1860), Cochrane patented the concept of using compressed air in tunnels and caissons, and Pol an Watelle of France discovered that the symptoms of decompression sickness could be relieved by recompression.

1860

In Oshwa, Canada, the first hyperbaric chamber on the North American continent was constructed for medical purposes.

1871

Paul Bert, a French scholar and politician, known as the Father of Pressure Physiology, proved that bubbles in the tissues during decompression were composed primarily of nitrogen. This finding was of more importance to the diving community than the medical community at the time, but it was an important step in saving the lives of divers. More importantly for hyperbaric medicine, it was Bert who built a chamber constructed entirely of technical devices he invented and built. He used his chamber primarily to scientifically demonstrate the toxic effect of hyperbaric oxygen on organisms. Bert was also the first to suggest that it might be best to use pure oxygen at atmospheric pressure for medical applications. This concept is the foundation of hyperbaric oxygen therapy used today.

1837 - 1877

"Pneumatic centers" (another term for hyperbaric centers) became popular in several European cities as a means for the wealthy to improve their health. Going to the pneumatic center for a treatment became as popular as going to the neighborhood gym is today. By 1877, there were many different types of chambers using compressed air in the major cities of Europe such as Berlin, Vienna, Amsterdam, Milan, London, and Brussels. The idea that pressurized air could improve one's health was spreading. Unfortunately, there was still no definitive information about how to run the chambers or who could be helped by the increased air tension. Neither were there any standardized procedures for administering the treatments. It was still left to the individual physician to use the treatments as he saw fit. Without any scientific proof as to the value of the chambers, many medical professionals became increasingly skeptical and recommended against using the chambers. Eventually, the public's interest in the chambers ebbed. The medical profession, as a whole, continued to view hyperbaric therapy as an experimental idea—maybe even a fad—without valid scientific documentation. About 30 - 40 years after the first chamber for "healthy" people was built, most of them closed because they were no longer economically viable.

1876

In the United States, a man named Daniel Kelly received a patent for a "Compressed Air Bath Apparatus." This was another chamber constructed for the well-being of the wealthy. Kelly's chamber was followed about 80 years later by a similar but more complex HBO chamber in Germany.

1885

The first known commercial use of hyperbaric chambers in North America occurred when tunnel workers, suffering from caisson's disease, were treated successfully in a recompression chamber. This was the invention of an English engineer, A.W. Moir, who also used the same concept to reduce deaths at the construction sites of tunnels in London. Although the treatments Moir used were highly successful and saved the lives of many of the workers who had become unconscious or paralyzed while working far underground, the physiological effects on the body were still unknown. For this reason, many in the scientific and medical communities found Moir's compressed air chambers as well as his rationale for the improvement of the construction workers hard to accept. The dramatic improvement in the health of the workers was proof that Moir's theories were correct, but he had no technology for proving his ideas.

1878

Another recommendation against the use of oxygen therapy was issued, this time by Paul Bert, because of the chance of toxicity. Instead, he advocated that normobaric air be used. Inasmuch as his experiments were primarily on animals, conducted in a small, riveted cylindrical vessel with a mechanically operated air compressor, it is not known how accurate his findings were. Nevertheless, his warning was enough to put another damper on the use of HBO in a medical setting.

1879

Fontaine, a French scientist, built a mobile pressure chamber with ten seats that was a great leap forward in its technical aspects. His chamber was used quite successfully as a mobile operating room. He, like his predecessors, showed amazing engineering skills and ideas that were far ahead of his time, but because he was unable to prove his theories about hyperbaric oxygen therapy they were not widely accepted.

1887

The first known book on hyperbaric medicine, written in 1887, contains more than 300 references to chambers and physicians who were studying the use of hyperbaric chambers for medical purposes in different parts of Europe and North America.

1891

Corning developed the first hyperbaric center in the United States; his intention was to treat patients with nervous disorders.

Early 1900s

As the commercial diving industry was beginning to develop, a great many different types of chambers were designed and used. By 1913, a German company had manufactured a chamber that could be folded and transported to areas where emergency treatments were needed for divers. In 1917, Dräger developed a system for treating diving incidents using oxygen under pressure. For reasons that are not clear, his system was never adopted.

The leader in hyperbaric chamber development in the United States during these times was Orville Cunningham. A physician with a brilliant engineering mind, he built his own gas-mixing machines to give his surgery patients more effective anesthesia, and was among the first to attempt to slow sound down to allow doctors to use a stethoscope to listen to heart activity. In both the hospital where he practiced and the medical school where he was a professor, he was greatly admired for his ability to diagnose illnesses and his surgical technical skills.

Among his many creative medical ideas, he thought that increased oxygenation might be effective against infections of various types. His ideas were based on the assumption that anaerobic infections play a role in the etiology of many diseases. He convinced the dean of the medical school in Kansas City, Missouri to give him permission to build a "tank" where he might conduct animal experiments. Before he could conduct these experiments, however, several patients dying of the Spanish flu were brought to him for a "last-ditch" treatment; all survived. Over the next few years, he built several small chambers. Not only did he help a great number of people survive the flu epidemic of the 1920s, but his treatments also helped others overcome medical problems for which traditional medicine was not effective.

It was not very long before people began to flock to Cunningham for treatments for a wide variety of illnesses. One of his most successful treatments was for diabetes mellitus. He also found that the new chambers were helpful in treating syphilis, a widespread medical problem for which there was no cure at the time. His medical colleagues from both the hospital and the medical school were impressed by Cunninghams's successes, but much to his consternation, did not embrace his compressed air theories. They thought he was profiting from unprofessional medical ideas. Cunningham to the contrary considered his actions to be highly ethical; he refused to advertise and did not like to have his name put in print.

In the March 5, 1921 issue of the *Saturday Evening Post*, an article entitled "What's Next in Science" said, without mentioning his name (at his request), "One of the most remarkable developments in recent times is the thought of using compressed air in the treatment of diseases that respond to increased oxidation."

Because of the word-of-mouth popularity of his work, Cunningham built larger chambers until he finally constructed the world's largest hyperbaric chamber in Cleveland, Ohio. This was completed in 1928 after he was forced to retire from the university and medical school because his colleagues were disappointed that he would not concentrate on "traditional" medical practices. The funds to build the Cleveland compressed air tank were given in gratitude by the Timken Bearing tycoon, 56-year-old Henry H. Timken, whose life had been saved by Cunningham. The round metal tank was five stories high and had 72 bedrooms, with the entire center furnished with items as luxurious as a first-class hotel. It was pressurized with compressed air and had a treatment sphere that could be pressurized to 2 ATA. As time went on, Cunningham's treatment pattern gradually changed and increased until the patient was placed under air pressure for one full week; this was followed by a week of rest, and then another full week of pressurization.

Cunningham's work was increasingly questioned by his own colleagues as well as the American Medical Association (AMA). AMA leaders became alarmed when Cunningham would not respond to their inquiries about what he was doing or why his treatments were medically sound. In 1928, he was formally censured by the AMA. Cunningham was either unwilling or unable to supply the scientific accounting demanded by the AMA. Gradually, the leaders of the AMA turned against him. They printed attacks on his professional ethics and techniques in their publications. This censure was quickly followed by the Cleveland Academy of Medicine which also questioned the validity of his work.

All of these attacks completely disregarded the fact that he had saved the lives of many patients with pneumonia and had treated a wide variety of other serious diseases. He had even had patients with positive serology for syphilis revert back to normal. Often, the dramatic results he achieved with patients occurred after all other known "traditional" medical treatments had failed.

Nevertheless, it was his fellow professionals who ostracized him to the extent that he spent the final part of his career working exclusively with his chambers. But according to his son, Cunningham felt the most important work he could do was to help sick people get well.

The economic condition of the country was his final enemy. In the days of the Depression, he was unable to borrow money to pay his bills. Money had become scarce even among his wealthiest patients, and business fell off. He was hounded by his creditors. Cunningham developed a serious heart condition, and was finally forced to sell the magnificent round, steel hospital to pay off his debts. He died at the age of fifty-seven. Inasmuch as he had never documented his successes or the treatments he had developed, the American Medical Association and the medical profession in general totally discounted his work. Sadly, Cunningham's million-dollar center, with his equipment inside, was dismantled for about $25,000 of scrap iron in 1942 to help the World War II effort. There is nothing left to show the ingenuity of this hyperbaric oxygen pioneer.

For the next decade, technical development and interest in hyperbaric chambers was confined to diving incidents rather than general medical applications.

1937

The modern age of hyperbaric medicine actually began in 1937, when Behnke and Shaw used a hyperbaric chamber to treat patients for decompression sickness. Still, interest lagged, and consensus on its medical value was widely divided. In the 1940s, the navy developed the first U.S. Navy Standard Treatment Tables. These became the standards for most of the world.

Another little known but major contributor to hyperbaric medicine as we know it today was Dr. Edgar End, M.D., of Milwaukee, Wisconsin. His first ventures into hyperbaric medicine came as a high school student when he and two friends constructed a diving helmet from a salvaged hot water tank, a piece of a motorcycle windshield, and some miscellaneous plumbing fixtures. When the young scientists were unable to get the device to submerge, they filled the pockets of an old overcoat with rocks. In this gear they descended into the murky green waters of a stone quarry.

End's next major experiment came in about 1942 after he had graduated from the Marquette University School of Medicine. He was asked by engineer and experienced diver Max Nohl to help improve Nohl's idea for an underwater breathing suit. Three cylinders were attached to the suit to allow the diver to rebreathe while removing carbon dioxide and replacing the oxygen. With this improved equipment, Nohl, aided by Dr. End, made a record dive of 420 feet to the bottom of Lake Michigan. Although these two young men were never recognized for this discovery, they had invented the first self-contained underwater breathing apparatus (scuba) outfit. This was the forerunner of Jacques Cousteau's aqua lung.

During World War II, End and his associates developed specialized equipment for the U.S. Navy, including frogman gear, underwater demolition team outfits, suits worn by disposal experts, and recirculation helmets.

During his career, End held more "firsts" in the field of underwater and hyperbaric medicine than any man in history. He was the first civilian to receive the Behnke Award of the Undersea Medical Society (the "Nobel Prize" of diving medicine). He also received the Simon Weisfeldt award in preventative medicine and was cited by the Milwaukee County Board for "contributions to medical knowledge and community health."

Among the discoveries made by this visionary of underwater and hyperbaric medicine was scientific proof that the inhalation of a helium-oxygen mixture, instead of compressed air, would free the deep sea diver from the narcotic effects of nitrogen and permit a more rapid decompression. This use of helium-oxygen is the basis for all modern deep sea diving.

End and his friend, Max Knohl, performed the first saturation dive and supervised world-record deep-dives in 1937 and 1942. In 1937, he also introduced the use of 100% oxygen at 3 ATA pressure to reduce the time required for decompression. He and Dr. Chester Long were the first to report successful treatment of carbon monoxide poisoning with hyperbaric oxygen in the experimental animal.

When End began treating victims of stroke and senility with hyperbaric oxygen in 1965, the results were startling. Some acute stroke victims were brought into his chamber unconscious and/or paralyzed and were able to walk out an hour later. According to an article in the *Milwaukee Medical Society Times*, Dr. End successfully treated patients afflicted with gas gangrene, chronic ulcer, precarious skin grafts, arteriosclerosis of the brain, migraines, and stroke. At this time, in addition to his private practice, he was an assistant clinical professor of environmental medicine at the Medical College of Wisconsin.

A myriad of divers, airmen, and patients owe Dr. End their lives for his belief in hyperbaric medicine. Unfortunately, for more than 40 years, he struggled to convince the rest of the establishment of the benefits of hyperbaric oxygenation. Like so many others before him, his work was not appreciated during his lifetime. Today, however, some of his applications of HBO are finally being accepted by the medical community.

1943

Jacques Cousteau improved on the scuba idea begun by End and Nohl and patented a device he called the aqua lung. Cousteau's excellent promotion of the aqua lung made deep diving much more accessible to recreational divers, and thus initiated a new wave of interest in hyperbaric medicine.

1947

A.R. Behnke discussed the main toxic effects of oxygen in his book *A Brief History of Hyperbaric Medicine*. In this book, he outlines information that must be understood in order to eliminate the possibility of oxygen toxicity:

1. The harmful effects of oxygen on the nervous system manifest themselves at pressures of 3 ATA and higher.
2. The nervous symptoms are concomitant with the elevation of oxygen tension in central venous blood.
3. Acidity of venous blood is increased.
4. Increasing the carbon dioxide tension in the lungs greatly enhances the toxicity of oxygen.
5. Adverse pulmonary and nervous system effects observed in man are reversible and are not followed by permanent gross injury.

Additional research by C.J. Lambersten found that toxicity could be further avoided if patients were treated at rest in a dry chamber. C. Fife and C. Piastadori concurred with these finding and reported in their review of oxygen toxicity that "Concern about oxygen toxicity should not restrict its use as a therapeutic modality when it may be clinically beneficial."

Nevertheless, the interest of the medical community in various types of medical treatments using hyperbaric oxygen therapy came to a virtual standstill for a few more years. It was not until after World War II that it became routine to use pressurized oxygen rather than pressurized air in hyperbaric chambers. In 1946, at a naval hospital, the U.S. Navy medical doctor George Hart used hyperbaric therapy to hasten wound healing. The patient was a young marine whose body metabolism was compromised to the point that his serious wounds would not heal properly. When the navy medical personnel saw the results of HBOT on the young marine, a new era in hyperbaric medical treatment began, with the military medical personnel leading the way. The techniques first developed by the military are now accepted medical practice for many types of wound healing.

1955

Not until 1955 was there any major interest in using HBO for other treatments. That year, Churchill-Davidson began to use oxygen therapy in a hyperbaric chamber to treat the damage suffered by cancer patients who have undergone radiation therapy. This was one of the first documented uses of pressurized oxygen rather than pressurized air as a medical treatment.

That same year, the man known as the Father of Modern HBO, Professor Ite Boerema, installed a large hyperbaric chamber in Amsterdam. In 1956, Boerema performed the first reported heart surgery in a hyperbaric chamber, and during the early 1960s he also began to treat patients with carbon monoxide intoxication and patients with vascular occlusions (blockage of blood vessels). Boerema also ran a group of experiments proving that when there is sufficient oxygen delivered to the tissues of animals, they can live temporarily without blood. He published his findings in medical journals in an article entitled "Life Without Blood." It was at this same hyperbaric center that W.H. Bummelkamp reported a successful treatment of gas gangrene in 1961. This is another widely accepted indication for HBOT today.

Despite the success of these experiments and procedures, the medical community on the whole was still reluctant to accept the concept that increased oxygenation would help cure or slow the progress of many diseases. The medical profession continued to discount hyperbaric oxygen therapy as a serious medical treatment in part because a group of unethical physicians in the 1960s began to "tout" hyperbaric oxygen treatments as a way to avoid the pitfalls of aging. These physicians promoted HBO treatments as a means of regrowing hair, increasing breast size, and improving virility. The public soon became disillusioned, and medical professionals cried "unethical" and "unproven." They were, of course, correct in this instance. Overall, using hyperbaric oxygen treatments did not maintain youth in its users, but it once again was a detriment to the acceptance of quality hyperbaric medicine for appropriate medicinal purposes.

1963 - 1973

HBO was shown to be effective in the management of osteomyelitis and for the early treatment in strokes during International Hyperbaric Conferences of 1963, '64, '65, '69, and '73. Some medical professionals were enthusiastic, but the average M.D. did not see the need for or the value of this new type of medicine. Others were still hesitant about the apparent dangers of using pressurized oxygen.

The Undersea Medical Society, U.S.A., was formed in 1967. The word "hyperbaric" was not added to their name until 1986, even though undersea workers who suffered diving incidents were the first to be treated on a regular basis using hyperbaric medicine. Today the Undersea Hyperbaric and Medical Society (UHMS) and the American College of Hyperbaric Medicine are leading organizations in this field. Hyperbaric physicians who belong to UHMS or the College should be well versed in hyperbaric medicine and have board certification.

HBO Around the World

The use of HBOT began in earnest in Germany in 1957, and between 1960 and 1970 a large number of monoplace and multiplace chambers were built. Most of these chambers used air for pressurization and pure oxygen under pressure via a mask. At that time there were no safety requirements for chambers, and the majority did not have a personal lock-up or oxygen delivery system although they could hold up to 28 people. Nevertheless, by 1976, Germany had approximately 30 centers where hyperbaric chambers were used for both diving and other medical purposes.

In other countries during the 1960s and 1970s, there was limited interest in the idea that pressurized oxygen could bring health to various parts of the body that were lacking oxygen. Russia, Austria, and Italy all had centers that started during this time period.

The belief that HBOT was medically sound began to grow. As early as 1964, studies published in the medical journal the *Lancet* demonstrated the positive effects of hyperbaric oxygenation on oxygen-deprived "blue babies." This was the first indication that it would be helpful in preventing cerebral palsy.

In 1987, K.K. Jain of Switzerland demonstrated the relief of spasticity in hemiplegia due to stroke by integrating HBO with physical therapy treatments while the patient was in the chamber.

In the 1990s, the number of countries that began studies about the effect of hyperbaric oxygen on children with cerebral palsy and serious head injuries grew rapidly. By the beginning of the year 2000, there were active chambers in South America, Japan, Cuba, China, Canada, the UK, France, Russia, Germany, Yugoslavia, and several other countries for treating a wide spectrum of medical conditions, including cerebral palsy.

Conclusion

The medical community owes a great deal to individuals who brought new ideas and procedures to the field of hyperbaric medicine. These founders of modern hyperbaric medicine were willing to stand apart from their fellow physicians and scientists and declare their belief in air and oxygen therapy. To demonstrate their faith in the new medical therapy, they used their ingenuity and intuition to design and construct chambers. They often suffered severe criticism from others and were ostracized by their fellow medical professionals. Clearly, without their belief in their own creative and innovative ideas, hyperbaric medicine might never have become available to treat so many of today's illnesses and diseases.

THE TEN QUESTIONS MOST OFTEN ASKED BY CAREGIVERS

Only the new smile of our daughter can tell the
story of how HBOT has changed our lives.

— Mrs. Yvette Serpelli
mother of one of the first
11 children in Canada to
undergo HBOT

Introduction

When considering a new form of therapy for a child with cerebral palsy or a traumatic brain injury, the burden of investigation and decision-making usually falls on the caregiver. Unfortunately, at this time, many physicians are not educated about hyperbaric medicine for this type of condition. The most effective method of obtaining the information that is needed to make an educated decision about the appropriateness of any type of therapy for a specific child is to ask questions. The ten questions most often posed by caregivers of children with cerebral palsy are listed in this chapter. Of course, these are very brief answers to quite complex questions. Listed at the end of each answer is the number of the chapter(s) where the specific topic is discussed in greater detail.

1. What is hyperbaric oxygen therapy (HBOT)?

It is a medical therapy that reduces cerebral edema (acute and long-term swelling) and improves the functions of the brain's tissues (neurons) that have been rendered inactive by ischemia / hypoxia (deficiency of oxygen) by giving 100% oxygen under pressure in a hyperbaric chamber. The improvement of brain function is reflected by the improved electrical activity of the brain. In other words, hyperbaric oxygen therapy (HBOT) is a medical treatment that uses pure oxygen under pressure to speed and enhance the body's natural ability to heal.

While sometimes used as a primary emergency treatment, it is more often used as a cost-effective adjunct of enhancement therapy for patients who suffer from various diseases or injuries associated with hypoxia (lack of oxygen) on a cellular level. It is at this cellular level where all life processes take place. (Chapters 1 and 3)

2. Is hyperbaric oxygen therapy safe for my child?

Under experienced medical supervision, HBOT is a safe, non-invasive form of therapy for children with cerebral palsy and brain injuries. It is important to remember, however, that the therapy should be given in a medical center under the direction of a trained hyperbaric medical physician, assisted by a trained, qualified staff. Like any other therapy modality, it can be unsafe when used by unqualified personnel or with improper equipment. (Chapter 8)

3. How soon will I see results?

This is a frequently asked question, but difficult to answer. We don't always see immediate improvement in children with cerebral palsy, but we often see rapid improvement in children with brain injuries. This is especially true if we treat the child soon after the brain damage occurs. In short, the sooner HBOT is started, the better the results. This often applies to the speed of improvement as well; the sooner the treatment is started after a brain injury of any type, the sooner improvements are observed. It appears that the longer the time that elapses before treatment is started, the longer it takes to see improvement and, to some degree, less improvement is seen. Furthermore, Dr. K.K. Jain in his *Textbook of Hyperbaric Medicine* reports that "repetitive HBO appears to be trophic, stimulatory to brain repair, and may not be complete in some cases until 200 - 300 treatments."

Of course, each child is different, as is the extent of his or her brain damage and its specific location. All of these factors affect the extent and rapidity of improvement.

Finally, one has to be realistic. Not all children see dramatic results. Sometimes the improvements are merely a decrease in the degree of spasticity, or the ability to hold a cup and drink with one hand rather than two hands. In other cases, the child is able to decrease or discontinue medication for seizures, or the frequency of seizures may diminish significantly. All of these improvements are important to the child and his or her caregiver, but may be difficult for an outsider to distinguish or to document scientifically. (Chapters 2 and 4)

4. What types of brain injuries does HBOT help?

As stated in the previous question, HBOT helps children in different ways. Cerebral palsy can be caused by many different injuries to the brain, including anoxia, infections, inoculations, traumas, etc., and every case is unique.

For example:
Eric was a healthy two-year-old until he fell, hit his head, slipped into the swimming pool, and nearly drowned. As a result of this accident and the beginning atrophy of his brain, a pediatric neurologist had predicted his outcome for recovery as zero. Just two months after his fall, he began receiving hyperbaric oxygen treatments. After 208 HBO treatments, he was vastly improved and had his life back. He continues to progress.

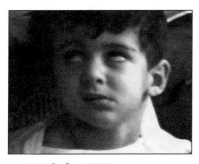 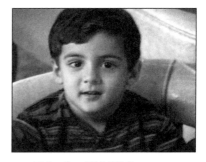

Eric before HBO   Eric after 208 HBO treatments

Amber was 14 years old and suffered from prolonged hypoglycemia because of diabetes and seizures. She was totally unresponsive and needed to be kept in a floor bed and fed through a tube in her nose. The only way she could stand up was with the help of three attendants. After 196 HBOT treatments she became much more self sufficient and was able to return to school.

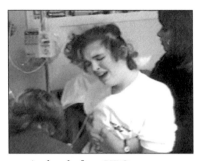

Amber before HBO

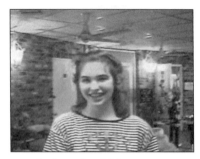

Amber after 196
HBO treatments

Jason was born with cerebral palsy that was diagnosed shortly after birth. At age 7, he had a vocabulary of 10 words and was still crawling to get around. After 61 HBO treatments, he was able to walk with help and had improved dramatically in his cognitive, vocal, and motor skills.

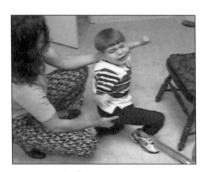

Jason before HBO

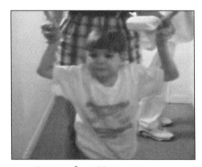

Jason after 61
HBO treatments

Alexandra was hit by a car and thrown 80 feet when she was an active 3-1/2-year-old. She was left unable to speak and was spastic in her right arm and her legs. After only 49 HBO treatments, she was walking, talking, and beginning to act like a curious, active 4-year-old. She has continued to make progress.

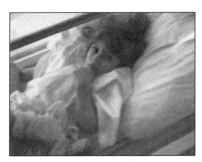

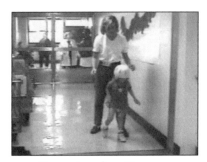

Alexandra before HBO   Alexandra after 49
                             HBO treatments

Regardless of whether brain injuries are traumatic (accidental) or vascular (stroke), or the result of a lack of oxygen during birth (hypoxia) or infections or vaccinations, all brain injuries have in common the destruction of brain cells and the formation of "idling" neurons. Diagnosis and treatment of the central nervous system requires the ability to distinguish between living and dead brain tissue.

5. Does it help every child?

Unfortunately, it doesn't. As with any medical intervention, there are some children who do not seem to improve significantly with hyperbaric oxygen treatments. For the most part, however, there is an 80 - 90% correlation between changes on the SPECT scan and noticeable improvement. Usually, this improvement can be determined before the child completes the initial 40 treatments, but not always. Occasionally, even when we do not see much change on the SPECT scans as the first series of treatments are concluding, parents will notice significant improvements later on. When the only change in the child's therapy is treatments in a hyperbaric chamber, it is difficult to discount the therapeutic value of HBOT. Once again, this is why each child must act as "his or her own control." (Chapter 6)

6. How many treatments will my child need?

Because each child is unique, the number of HBOT treatments will vary. The actual number of treatments will depend, in part, on age, health, speed of improvement, goal of treatments, caregivers' time frame, financial means, etc.

Each case is very different, but at this time standard protocol is to give an initial series of 40 - 80 treatments unless a different number is needed, depending on the medical reason for the treatment. Each treatment will last approximately an hour, with time of treatment starting from the moment that the chamber begins to be pressurized. Most often, there may be a break between treatment series of as much as a year; the time frame of the sets of treatments (referred to as doses) is based upon when the treatments are started as well as family logistics and finances. Longer term conditions take more time to correct. Certain patients have had over 300 treatments with continuing improvement. (Chapter 6)

7. What is a SPECT scan? How does it work?

The word SPECT stands for single photon emission computerized tomography. It is a scan of the brain that documents the functional actions of the brain in much the same way as MRIs, x-rays, and EKGs document the anatomy of other parts of the body. With HBOT, the SPECT is used pre HBOT to develop a baseline of how the brain is functioning. Periodic additional SPECT scans are used to determine if and to what degree activity in the neurons has increased.

The SPECT scan has the power to identify and provide a digital image of brain function. Although there are other diagnostic imaging systems available, the SPECT scan is the most practical and widely accepted diagnostic procedure used in conjunction with HBOT.

An increasing number of studies have verified that SPECT imaging with interventional hyperbaric oxygen therapy is useful in locating recoverable brain tissue in injuries caused by oxygen deprivation. The data supplied by the use of the SPECT scan supports the hypothesis that traumatic, vascular, and anoxic brain injuries as well as those caused by infections and toxicity all have a common pathology which includes the possibility of recoverable brain cells. The SPECT scan is obtained by using a gamma camera and a minimal amount of an isotope injected into the arm or hand. (Chapter 6)

8. How can I choose a well-run center?

There are between 500 and 700 HBOT chambers in the United States. Many of these chambers are used exclusively for diving incidents or for testing and training divers with simulated depths. Other chambers are in hospitals or centers that do not provide HBO treatments to children with cerebral palsy or brain injuries on a regular basis. Often these hyperbaric centers in hospitals are used exclusively for the 14 treatments currently authorized by Medicare. In some cases, a hospital may choose not to use the hyperbaric chamber for head injuries or illnesses in children because the physician(s) in charge prefers to "wait and see."

There are four primary elements to look for in a qualified hyperbaric center:

1. *Staff qualifications* – in addition to the hyperbaric physician who evaluates each patient and his or her respective SPECT scans, the rest of the staff should be experienced in the use of hyperbaric chambers and trained in the process and procedures of treating children with increased oxygen tension.

2. *Properly equipped facility* – to make certain that the child receives the correct amount of oxygen, it is important that the hyperbaric chambers be properly constructed and maintained. There are many different types and shapes of hyperbaric chambers, but the two most often used for HBOT in cases of children with cerebral palsy or brain injuries are the monoplace (single person) or the multiplace (2 - 12 people). Each of these chambers has advantages and disadvantages; the proper chamber will depend on the child, the cause of the brain injury, and the number of treatments that are needed. (Chapter 7)

3. *Primary focus of the center* – it is advantageous to the health and welfare of the individual using the hyperbaric chamber to receive HBO treatments where the primary focus of the center is treatment of neurological problems. If the hyperbaric chamber is an adjunct to some other type of business or medical service, or has a focus on other types of hyperbaric services such as wound healing, it may be that the medical procedures for children with cerebral palsy or head injuries could be compromised by placing these children in a multiplace chamber where other pressures are utilized. Protocols for children with cerebral palsy or traumatic brain injuries are entirely different than protocols used for other medical conditions.

4. *System for documenting need and result of the treatments* – it is critical that the center have an approved method of documenting the necessity of HBO treatments and the results achieved. As has been noted, some children may not respond well to HBO treatments

because of the condition of their brain damage, its location, or the absence of idling neurons. It is also important to confirm that the treatment are remedying the damaged areas by doing periodic SPECT scans. (Chapter 6)

9. How far advanced is HBO research in the United States?

HBO therapy is still considered an alternative therapy in the U.S. It will remain in this alternative status until controlled, double-blind studies are conducted. In other countries, it is possible to do controlled studies with funding provided by the government. In the United States, most of the funding for neurological studies is regulated by the National Institute of Neurological Disorders and Strokes (NINDS), operated under the auspices of the United States Department of Health and Human Services (which is part of the National Institutes of Health). As of this time, HHS has not allocated money for this type of study, and the cost of controlled, double-blind studies in the U.S. is approximately $250,000 each.

In addition, studies on new procedures, medications, or protocols are usually funded in the United States by pharmaceutical companies where profit must be the primary focus. Pressurized oxygen is not a "drug" that pharmaceutical companies find financially advantageous.

Finally, most medical schools do not have courses on hyperbaric medicine as part of their standard curriculum. As of now, only 12 - 15 of the many medical schools in the U.S. have a course in hyperbaric medicine. This lack of training does not give the average physician a comprehensive understanding of hyperbaric medicine or the knowledge needed to assist caregivers to make an informed decision about its use.

10. Why doesn't my doctor recommend it?
**   Why won't my insurance pay for it?**

There are a variety reasons why a doctor may not recommend HBOT. The primary reasons are these:

1. As stated earlier, hyperbaric medicine is not taught in most medical schools in the United States at this time. Consequently, your doctor may not know much about it.
2. There are limited controlled, double-blind studies proving that this treatment should no longer be considered an alternative therapy and

that it should be listed as a viable therapy for children with cerebral palsy and brain injuries.

3. Neither the federal government's Health Department, NINDS, nor the primary cerebral palsy associations have taken a firm stand for or against this type of therapy. They do warn that the results have not yet been proven, but they acknowledge that the treatment may be helpful.

4. Cerebral palsy is not yet among the 14 conditions that have been formally approved by the American Medical Association or Medicare and for which Blue Cross / Blue Shield and many other private insurance companies now pay.

The National Institute of Health (NIH) in the United Kingdom is now paying for treatments for children with cerebral palsy, but in the U.S. the majority of insurance companies do not typically pay for treatments that have not been formally approved by either Medicare or the AMA. There are a few progressive companies that have begun to cover HBOT for the brain-injured child, but as long as HBOT for cerebral palsy is considered alternative, treatment costs will remain the responsibility of the caregiver.

On the positive side, most major insurance companies will pay for the medical evaluation of the child, including the SPECT scans, both for diagnostic purposes to begin treatment and subsequent scans to document improvement to brain function as well as necessary concomitant therapies.

State and federal legislation have been important tools in gaining acceptance in the United States for HBOT as a therapy for the brain-injured child. For example, legislation has recently been passed in Texas approving the use of hyperbaric oxygen treatments for anyone with cognitive dysfunction. This is, however, a general term, and although the law is in effect, the actual utilization is not clear. The state of California is also in the process of seeking approval for the use of HBOT in cases of children with cerebral palsy and brain-injuries. Furthermore, Virginia, West Virginia, North Carolina, South Carolina, and Missouri have all reimbursed HBOT for brain-injured children, and the states of Alaska, Arkansas, and Florida have indicated that they will change their policy decisions. Perhaps most significantly, a court decision in Georgia overturned Georgia Medicaid's denial of HBOT. This court decision could be used as a model in other states. All of these events mark progress toward bringing HBOT into the realm of accepted therapies for children with cerebral palsy and brain injuries.

Summary

By including not only the rationale of HBOT, but also its history, pertinent research, and physiological effects of oxygen on the body, specifically on the brain, it is hoped that caregivers will feel more confident about making their own decisions about the value of hyperbaric oxygen therapy for their child. It is important for the caregiver to remember that like any other form of therapy, HBOT is not intended to be the exclusive treatment used in cases of children with cerebral palsy or brain injuries. Rather, it is recommended that it be part of the overall plan to help the child obtain as much independence and normal body function as possible. It is further hoped that members of the healthcare team, including physical, occupational, and speech therapists, will view HBOT as an ally to the individual child's plan of care.

This book was designed to be used in whatever way the caregiver feels it will be of most benefit. Caregivers should have access to the information they need to talk objectively to their own physician and care-giving team about this treatment modality. Each reader should feel confident about the choices he or she makes concerning hyperbaric oxygen therapy.

POSITIVE EFFECTS OF HYPERBARIC OXYGENATION IN CERTAIN MITOCHONDRIAL CYTOPATHIES

All life takes place on a cellular level. This is the first
scientific proposal that hyperbaric oxygenation may
selectively turn mitochondrial genes on and off.
—Richard A. Neubauer, M.D.

Introduction

The simplest life on earth as we know it occurs in cells. Over the millennia, as cells evolved into more complex organisms, the new life depended upon the integrated and coordinated activities of thousands, millions, and even billions of cells, each one requiring appropriate oxygen and glucose for respiration, metabolism, production of energy, adaptation, reproduction, and overall survival.

For cells to carry out their unique functions, they require a variety of foods with which to build their various cellular structures, as well as their unique proteins, lipids, and carbohydrates, and from which the cells extract the energy to carry on all their vital activities.

The energy is derived in a series of biochemical reactions, which involves the burning of sugar (glucose) in the foods animals eat with the oxygen they breathe. Normally when animals living on land, including humans, take a deep breath, they inhale air containing 19–21% oxygen. From here on we will limit the discussion to humans, keeping in mind that similar activities, with variations in the details, also occur in other living organisms, especially mammals, the group of organisms to which humans belong.

The inhaled oxygen is not only dissolved in the bloodstream, but it also binds to a molecule in the red blood cell called hemoglobin. The dissolved and bound oxygen is then transported through all of the blood vessels down to the tiniest capillaries. The bound oxygen is released and, along with the dissolved oxygen, diffuses to the individual cells of tissues and organs. Then the carbon dioxide produced by the metabolism of the cells is bound to the hemoglobin and transported to the lungs for elimination from the body.

The Amazing Experiment

Before discussing the transport of oxygen and its utilization by the cells, it is important to note that if the circulation is blocked, such as it is in gangrene, myocardial infarction (heart attack), or in stroke, the consequences are deleterious. Even small reductions in blood flow will reduce the delivery of oxygen to the tissues and organs. In 1960, Dr. Ite Boerema of Holland took a group of pigs from a farm and removed every drop of blood from them. He then substituted an artificial blood plasma to keep the circulation working and the heart pumping, and put them into a hyperbaric chamber. Under hyperbaric oxygen conditions, even without a drop of blood, every organ functioned normally. Being frugal, he re-transfused half of the pigs and returned them to the farm. The other half were subjected to organ examination. Even with the total lack of blood there were no abnormalities in any organ: heart, lung, brain, kidneys, spleen, or bone. This was an extremely important observation and showed clearly that life could be supported in a mammal without blood (red blood cells). This remarkable observation was very influential in the development of the field of hyperbaric medicine. It also introduced the use of hyperbaric oxygen as a substitute for blood transfusion to Jehovah's Witnesses.

Let us now return to the release of oxygen from the hemoglobin in the capillaries. Each step in the process of transporting oxygen to cells is important. The last step, the breaking off of the oxygen from the hemoglobin and its subsequent diffusion to the cells and their utilization of it, is very important. It is at these last stages that the cells are going to use the oxygen to convert the energy from glucose into a chemical compound that drives the life processes. This last step is energy-laden.

The Cells

Cells are the building blocks of all living organisms. Each cell has a center, called the nucleus, which contains the genetic information for the building, repairing, and functioning of the cells. The rest of the cell, the material outside the nucleus to the edge of the cell (the cell membrane), is called the cytoplasm (the liquid-gel portion of the cell). The cytoplasm contains essential sub-cellular structures (organelles), one of the most important being the mitochondria, where energy is obtained in a form that can be utilized by the cell.

The Chromosomes

The nucleus of every human cell (except the mature red blood cells, which have no nucleus) contains 46 chromosomes (23 pairs); one chromosome of each pair is derived from each parent. The only other exception to the 23-pair distribution is the reproductive cells. The male sperm and female egg each contain 23 chromosomes. During fertilization, one of the chromosomes from the mother pairs up with its corresponding chromosome from the father to produce a cell containing 23 pairs of chromosomes. Twenty-two pairs are autosomal chromosomes and one pair is the sex chromosomes. Each chromosome contains genes which direct the growth, development, and function of the human body.

The Genes

The genes, located on the chromosomes, are the basic units of heredity. One of the major functions of genes is to direct the synthesis of proteins. Thus, genes create proteins and proteins create us. Proteins are formed on the instructions found within the specific genes and consist primarily of amino acids. Proteins are the body's workhorses, carrying out chemical structural function within the cells and, on higher levels of biological complexity, tissues and organs. Like DNA and RNA (to be discussed below), proteins are three-dimensional. A faulty gene can create a misshapen protein which, in turn, alters its function.

DNA and RNA

Genes are composed of a complex chemical called deoxyribonucleic acid (DNA). DNA is the chemical basis of genetics and heredity. DNA is in the form of a double helix molecule which encodes the unique genetic blueprint of cells' individual traits. DNA is composed of four compounds called nucleotides. These nucleotides consist of two purine- and two pyrimidine-containing compounds. The purines are adenine (A) and guanine (G), and the pyrimidines are thymine (T) and cytosine (C). These four compounds fit together in a special way: The A always pairs with T. The G pairs with C. Any disarrangement of this complex puzzle may represent a misspelling of the message, thereby sending wrong instructions to the cell, leading to a miswired development or function.

Every human baby is 99.9% identical in DNA makeup to every other human baby. It is the slightest deviation of only 0.1% that makes us unique individuals. In fact we are 98% identical in DNA to the great apes (chimpanzees). Even after billions of years of evolution we are 97% identical to the DNA in the yeast molecule. From comparative physiology and biochemistry we learn that what occurs in other organisms, especially on the molecular level of biologic organization, may well occur in other living species as well. Thus, studies in yeast could profoundly influence our understanding of what happens in mammals, including humans.

RNA (ribonucleic acid) is an information-encoded strand of nucleotides similar to DNA but with two slight changes: one of the pyrimidines, thymine, is replaced by a different one, uracil, and deoxyribose is replaced by a different five-carbon sugar, ribose. DNA needs RNA in order to carry out its instructions. There are several types of RNA, each with a slightly different function. For example, mRNA (messenger RNA) mediates between DNA and proteins, while tRNA (transfer RNA) works to line up the amino acids correctly. These amino acids are bound together to form proteins. The process of protein synthesis occurs in cellular organelles called ribosomes. Ribosomes are composed of protein and a third kind of RNA, rRNA (ribosomal RNA).

Genes are composed of segments of long DNA molecules which have their sequences transcribed onto messenger RNA, which then serves as a template for protein synthesis. Basically, DNA codes for the structure of messenger RNA, and mRNA codes for the structure of the specific proteins. Each gene is responsible for the structure of a specific protein.

In the 1990s, another type of RNA, microRNA, was discovered. (The basic structure of DNA had not even been discovered until 1953.) MicroRNA is a very short and unusual piece of RNA. Instead of synthesizing proteins, this tiny molecule latches onto messenger RNA, causing its destruction. Without messenger RNA no protein is produced.

In effect, the gene for that particular protein has been silenced. MicroRNA was originally thought to be an oddity or anomaly in a single species but has now been identified in various plants and animals—200 in humans alone.

Protein production is a highly regulated process. The process of turning a gene on or off, depending on the cell's need for a particular protein, is called regulation of gene expression. Gene regulation is an essential part of life and is also critical for cellular response to metabolic needs. Since every cell in an organism contains the same genetic blueprint, different cell types are created by turning on and turning off different genes at different times during development. It is gene expression that allows stem cells to become unique cell types by being turned on ("expressed") or off ("silenced") in just the right combinations, resulting in stem cells producing either heart cells, bone cells, or brain cells, etc. The discovery of microRNA helps us to begin to understand these complex biological processes. It is now suspected that silencing particular genes at just the right times—a process called RNA interference—will push genetically identical cells down different paths of development, enabling some to perceive light while others digest food.

One of the important areas of research in modern biochemistry and developmental biology is learning about conditions and factors that turn genes on and off. In yeast, it has been learned that oxygen is one of these factors.

The Mitochondria and Energy Synthesis

Oxygen is utilized in the cell primarily in the organelle called a mitochondrion (singular). Cells have many mitochondria (plural), depending on the specific function(s) of the cells and the amount of energy they require to carry out their functioning. Mitochondria are essential to every cell in the body. In 1963, it was discovered that mitochondria even contain their own genetic material (mtDNA) which is separate from the genetic material found in the cell nucleus (nDNA). Mitochondria are responsible for processing oxygen and converting the energy stored in the chemical structure of the foods we eat into a form that cells can use as a driving force for all essential cell functions. Energy is produced in the form of a chemical compound called adenosine triphosphate (ATP).

ATP is the universal currency of energy for all living organisms—i.e., all living organisms convert the energy in food to ATP. ATP is transported from the mitochondria to the cytoplasm (the liquid-gel portion of a cell) for its use in multiple cell functions.

Mitochondrial Diseases

Mitochondrial diseases—now known as mitochondrial cytopathies— vary in clinical conditions depending upon the disturbance in the genetic makeup of the mitochondria. Much information has been discovered since the 1940s and 1950s, when the first patient was diagnosed with a mitochondrial disease. Currently, there are over 40 known (identified) mitochondrial cytopathies. The main factor among these diseases is that the mitochondria are unable to completely burn the food with oxygen in order to generate sufficient energy (ATP) to sustain the integrated and coordinated functions of the cells, and thereby the functions of tissues and organs. These processes require numerous chemical reactions, all exquisitely coordinated, in order to have a continuous supply of energy to sustain life.

Incompletely burned food that accumulates may act as (a) poison(s) inside the body. These poisons can stop other chemical reactions that are essential for cell survival, making the energy crisis worse. In addition, some of these poisons can act as free radicals, highly reactive chemicals which readily form harmful compounds with other molecules. Free radicals can damage the mitochondrial DNA, which has very limited repair abilities.

Mitochondrial diseases are classified according to the organ systems affected and the symptoms that are present. In certain cases, only one organ is involved, while in other patients multiple organs may be affected, and each system may have a wide variance of dysfunction. Depending upon how severe the mitochondrial disorder is, the illness may range in severity from mild to fatal. Mitochondrial cytopathies may affect any system of the body from the brain to the eyes, ears, gastrointestinal system, muscles, heart, liver, pancreas, thyroid, immune system, etc., or any combination of the above. This essentially creates an infinite number of manifestations of mitochondrial disease.

In the United States, approximately 4,000 children have been diagnosed with or have developed mitochondrial diseases by the age of ten.

Between 1,000 and 4,000 children per year are born with some type of mitochondrial disease in the US.

Many diseases of aging have also been found to cause defects in mitochondrial function in adults, including, but not limited to, Type II diabetes, Parkinson's disease, artherosclerosis, heart disease, stroke, Alzheimer's, and cancer. It must be noted that many medications and toxins may injure mitochondrial function at any stage of life. In many patients, mitochondrial disease may be an inherited condition, i.e., it runs in families (genetic), with an uncertain percentage of patients acquiring symptoms due to other factors.

Types of Mitochondrial Disease Inheritance: Autosomal Recessive Inheritance

Autosomal recessive inheritance may be the most common of the mitochondrial disorders. Remember that we all have two copies of every gene: one from our mother and one from our father. Only one of the two genes randomly enters an egg or sperm as it is formed. One gene from both egg and sperm results in the baby having two copies of that gene. In autosomal recessive inheritance, both parents are carriers of the defective gene, but they each have only one copy. The parents are not affected because they also have a normal copy of the same gene. If both the egg and sperm carry the defective (bad, mutant) gene, then the child will have no working (normal) copies and will thereby manifest the disorder. Autosomal recessive inherited mitochondrial disorders usually result in severe disease with infantile onset.

Therefore, there is only a 25% chance that a child will inherit the defective gene from both parents and manifest the disease (the same percentage applies to other siblings). Fifty percent of the children will inherit the defective gene from only one parent and will become unaffected carriers (like their parents), and 25% of the children will not inherit either copy of the defective gene.

Autosomal Dominant Inheritance

With dominant inheritance, only one copy of the defective gene is required in order for the associated disorder to develop; any child that inherits the defect should theoretically manifest symptoms of the disease. Occasionally this may not occur. In children who do show symptoms of the disease, the severity can vary markedly. Both autosomal recessive and autosomal dominant inheritance are similar in regards to the highly variable manifestations of the problems caused by the defective gene. If the trait is dominant, however, there is a 50% chance of it occurring in other siblings.

Maternal Inheritance

Both male and female children inherit their mitochondrial DNA (mtDNA) only from their mother, unlike the inheritance of nuclear DNA, which comes from both the mother and the father. Maternally inherited mitochondrial disorders are not rare and possibly are as common as autosomal recessive inherited disorders. All mitochondrial disorders are maternally inherited.

While each of our cells contain exactly two copies of virtually every nuclear gene, each cell contains varying numbers of mtDNA copies, often several thousand per cell. People with maternally inherited mitochondrial disease may have any number of defective mtDNA cells. While one might assume that the more mutant mtDNA a cell contains, the more problems it will have, actually the cell works quite well until the proportion of mutant mtDNA reaches a threshold (which varies among different tissues and by the nature of the different mutations). Since there is a 100% chance of the trait occurring in other siblings, mtDNA inheritance has a more serious prognosis for the family than autosomal inheritance, although the effects may be more or less severe. This means that the symptoms, severity, age of onset, etc., may vary tremendously within a family. Again, such variations could create an almost infinite number of manifestations. Unlike autosomal recessive inheritance, the onset of maternally inherited disorders is usually seen somewhat later in life, with the manifestations occurring anywhere from toddler age well into adulthood.

The combination of mtDNA and nDNA defects and their correlation in mitochondrial formation and function is as yet unknown.

At times, the diagnosis of mitochondrial disease is extremely evasive and invasive, not to mention time and labor intensive, and in most cases extremely expensive. A single muscle biopsy may cost in the range of $26,000, so many insurance providers refuse to reimburse for this potentially important and powerful diagnostic technique, especially when it may require multiple biopsies for a specific diagnosis to be obtained. Some doctors and/or medical centers may even be unwilling to recommend this testing, since all mitochondrial diseases are thought to be untreatable and are lump-summed into a vague category of incurable disorders for which the only treatment options are to try to ameliorate some of the symptoms, keep the patient comfortable, and/or to perhaps delay or prevent progression of the disease. Current treatment usually involves intensive vitamin and enzyme therapies, along with occupational and physical therapy. The rationale seems to be that it is not worth the time, trouble, or expense to specifically identify a disease which the medical community basically has no idea how to treat. Unfortunately, from a variety of perspectives, diagnosis thereby becomes irrelevant and unnecessary. It is often due to the parents' tenacity in pursuit of a definitive diagnosis that the more intensive tests are performed.

It is usually the "ruling-out" of the obvious simple causes of multiple, often extremely serious symptoms that finally initiates the quest for a diagnosis of a possible mitochondrial disorder. Sometimes problems are noted by almost every doctor the child visits, i.e., neurologist, pediatrician, ophthalmologist, or orthopedic specialist, etc. However, these observations may never be brought together into a coherent theory of diagnosis. It is especially true in the evaluation of the infant or child with the possible risk of mitochondrial disease that medicine should not be "cubby-holed" by specialty. It is therefore urged that parents discuss all aspects of their child's health with each medical professional; mention your child's change in vision or bowel/bladder habits to your child's neurologist and the opthalmologist's or gastroenterologist's concerns to your neurologist or pediatrician. Hopefully, by so doing, you will be giving them all a path of discovery into your child's problem.

Just as in any medical evaluation, diagnosis of mitochondrial disease begins simply with a family history and physical/neurological examination of the patient. From that point, metabolic examinations will include blood, urine, and spinal fluid tests (if necessary). If there is neurologic involvement, testing should include SPECT brain imaging to ascertain brain blood flow/metabolism or magnetic resonance imaging (MRI) to determine anatomic problems in the brain. Retinal or electroretinogram might be ordered for detection of a visual disorder and

EKG (echocardiogram) might be called for if cardiologic symptoms are present. Evoked potentials, which measure the nerve conduction from the brain back and forth to the eyes (VEP: visual evoked potentials) and the ears (BAER: brain auditory evoked response), may also need to be tested. Blood tests may be needed to determine thyroid function and also to perform genetic DNA testing. The more invasive tests, such as biopsy of skin, muscle, or brain, are, as stated earlier, invasive and expensive, and are only performed as needed.

In this chapter we present one of the most complex mitochondrial disorders ever described with a totally remarkable outcome resulting from hyperbaric oxygen therapy. This is the case of little Gracie.

Gracie

Mitochondrial cytochrome c reductase deficiency is an extremely rare condition. Only five cases ever diagnosed and cited in medical reviews worldwide could be found. Life expectancy is considered to be virtually zero. In four of the cases identified, the children died as infants (at < 15 months). The fifth case is Gracie.

Gracie spent the first year and a half of her life in hospitals, being flown all over the country, at an expenditure of over $10 million dollars. She eventually had over 15 biopsies, including tissue samples taken from brain, muscle, and rectum. Gracie's final diagnosis was that she had a disorder of oxidative phosphorylation, a mitochondrial function. The intense vitamin therapy program which allowed her to survive as long as she had consisted of 16 vitamins that were given every two hours, and cost $4,000 per month.

When first seen at the Ocean Hyperbaric Neurologic Center (03/28/02), Gracie was three years old, weighed 11 pounds, and was diagnosed "failure to thrive." She was in a vegetative-like state, blind from optic atrophy, G-tube dependent, hypotonic, speechless, unable to crawl, and unable to sit up, and she lacked both fine and gross motor control. She had seizures and central apnea. Gracie had no sensation to pain and did not respond to touch or voice. There was severe cognitive deficit, and she was physically and developmentally at an infant (three months) stage.

Although we had never treated a case of this disorder (there being no other survivors), HBO is known to increase O_2 availability to the mitochondria and to have a positive effect on cytochrome c oxidase function when used as the primary treatment for severe carbon monoxide intoxication. On these theoretical bases, we agreed to attempt a trial of hyperbaric oxygen treatments for Gracie.

Prior to the initiation of hyperbaric oxygen therapy, a baseline SPECT brain scan was obtained at an independent institution (see Figs. 1–3). It showed a severe anoxic ischemic encephalopathy (AIE). This neurologic aspect of Gracie's condition had never been diagnosed before (as every other aspect of her health seemed to take precedence over concern with her brain function). Since hyperbaric oxygen treatments are a principle treatment of AIE, they were started immediately. Gracie's gradual physical improvement following 20 hyperbaric oxygen treatments was correlated with an improvement in her April 2002 repeat brain SPECT scan done at Joe DiMaggio's Children's Hospital in Hollywood, Florida. The radiologist's report states: "There has been a dramatic improvement in the appearance of the perfusion pattern to the brain."

Over a two month period, Gracie received 63 hyperbaric oxygen treatments (1 hour at 1.5 ATA), and she began making surprisingly rapid developmental progress. She began to use her hands meaningfully. She learned to not only sit upright but to hold her balance and could pull up in her crib to standing. She began to say "Mama," "baba," and other meaningful vocalizations. She passed her swallow study; all nutrition was now being taken orally, and she began to eat solid foods. The medications she was on for seizures, reflux, and mitochondrial patterns were being tapered off. The intense vitamin program was no longer necessary, as her body began to maintain these levels naturally, thus saving the family over $28,000 (to date). All visual impairment disappeared, and she began to see things and reach for them. A pivotal moment, says her mom, was when the family was at a Greek restaurant and everyone began to throw plates to celebrate the ambience after the meal. Gracie actually reached out for a plate, grabbed it, and threw it onto the floor like everyone else (with great delight, it might be added). Subsequently, two independent ophthalmologists confirmed no evidence of optic atrophy and confirmed that she now appeared to be, at least visually, a normal child. Hyperbaric oxygen treatments were continued. Final SPECT scans after 235 treatments (2/10/03) showed dramatic improvement with a complete normalization of all previous perfusion/metabolism deficits.

On March 20, 2003, after 238 treatments, Gracie's feeding tube was removed. Gracie was on her way to a more normal life. The hyperbaricist and pediatric intensivist were of the opinion that with continued hyperbaric oxygen treatment and intensive physical, occupational, and speech therapy, Gracie could reach limits never thought or dreamed possible.

Another muscle biopsy taken after 242 HBOT treatments (5/11/03) confirmed that Gracie's muscle showed no evidence of cytochrome c reductase deficiency. As stated on the report by Georgirene D. Viadutiu, Ph.D., at Buffalo Children's Hospital:

No abnormalities were found among the enzymes analyzed. Succinate cytochrome c reductase moved from 14% in the respiratory chain to 82%. Medical genetics report states, "Dramatic significant developmental achievements in the last 3 months coincident with treatment of hyperbaric oxygen therapy."

An important component of any assessment of the therapeutic efficacy, especially in young children, should include its impact on the family: This is what Gracie Kenitz's family had to say:

Hyperbaric oxygen therapy has changed our whole life. We will be forever grateful for the people who believed that Gracie should live, and who supported us in a decision that so many physicians were against.

We have seen so many changes in Gracie's life—ones we only dreamed of and never thought possible. Gracie is catching up daily in her developmental milestones. She now responds to touch, voices and music. Our older daughter, Lily, now has a sister she can grow up with, and Gracie has grandparents who can spoil her, a father who looks to the day he can teach her to drive and someday walk her down the aisle on her wedding day. We are indebted to Dr. Raul Ponte, Grace's pediatric intensivist from St. Mary's Hospital, for stepping out of the role of modern medicine and telling us to try HBOT when most of his collegues were against it, and to our hero, Dr. Richard A. Neubauer, who is not only an exceptional physician, but an extraordinary human being who gave us a glimpse of hope when so many others did not.

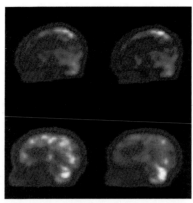

Figure 1. SPECT scans of Gracie's brain pre-treatment (top) and post-treatment (bottom).

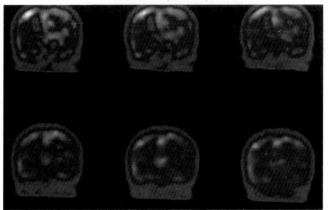

Figures 2. SPECT scans of Gracie's brain pre-treatment (top) and post-treatment (bottom).

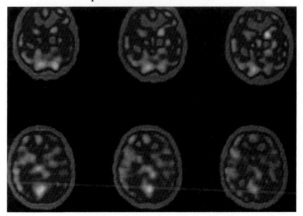

Figures 3. SPECT scans of Gracie's brain pre-treatment (top) and post-treatment (bottom).

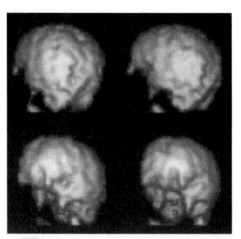

Figure 4. Pre-treatment SPECT scan of Brooke's brain.

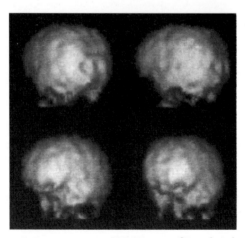

Figure 5. Post-treatment SPECT scan of Brooke's brain.

Because of HBOT our daughter can now laugh, smile, and play—the three things that are so vital to childhood remembrance. HBOT gave us the opportunity to be a complete family again, to look into the future with hope and dreams instead of confusion and sadness. We now don't recall what we missed and lost with her in her first three years, but rather what we have gained from her, such as unconditional love and joy and a future with unlimited possibilities. Grace is now age five and has had 384 hyperbaric oxygen treatments. On August 23, 2004, Grace will start kindergarten.

Summer

Summer was four years old when first seen in April of 2004. She was delivered at 36 weeks and stopped breathing twice during the process. At birth she was apneic (hypoxic). At one year of age she had 39 seizures in three days and developed apnea. The seizures started on one side of the head and progressed to the other. She finally had three types of seizures: grand mal, shuddering, and staring. The mother was told at this time that Summer had heart defects and a liver abnormality. Summer ate a normal diet but remained very thin. She was given a working diagnosis of Angelman's disease. It remains highly frustrating to the family to later find out that the symptoms for Angelman's and Leigh's diseases are almost identical, and that Summer's pattern of symptoms perfectly fit both diagnoses. Yet she was only tested for one (Angelman's), and it was over a year later that she was finally tested and diagnosed with Leigh's. It was not until she was two years old that they could even arrange for the biopsy to discern the ultimate answer. The final diagnosis of Leigh's was made by a single muscle biopsy sent to Horizon Molecular in Atlanta in 2002.

Leigh's disease is a rare inherited neurometabolic disorder characterized by degeneration of the central nervous system caused by either mutations in the mitochondrial DNA or by deficiencies of an enzyme called pyruvate dehydrogenase. Symptoms usually begin between the ages of three months to two years and progress rapidly. The first signs may be poor sucking ability and loss of head control and motor skills and may be accompanied by continuous crying, vomiting, loss of appetite, and seizures. Symptoms may later include generalized weakness, lack of muscle tone, and episodes of lactic acidosis, which can lead to impairment of kidney and respiratory function. Leigh's disease can also begin during late adolescence or early adulthood and progress more slowly.

It was initially thought that Summer might be developmentally delayed, although she could say over 45 words. The family had even started teaching her how to feed herself and drink from a regular cup, but within a two month period all of this progress disappeared. She could suddenly no longer feed herself, nor could she say a word. It was postulated that her brain processing had stopped and that she might from now on simply mumble a few words now and then. The doctors now felt that there was no hope and that her life expectancy would be 5–7 years. They told the mother that Summer would need a g-tube and trach and would probably die at home. The records showed that she was also diagnosed with atrial septal defect and ventricular portal ductus arteriosis. The mother was told that the mitochondrial disease would attack every part of Summer's body.

When seen at the Ocean Hyperbaric Neurologic Center, Summer's medical evaluation noted hypotonia, particularly in the hips and the legs, although she was very mobile and active. The heart defects had been surgically repaired in Atlanta. A VSD patch was in place, and the cardiologist said that the leakage associated with the patch would eventually heal itself. A year prior to being seen at OHNC it was thought that she was having "break-through" seizures. Summer was hospitalized for a 48-hour EEG, yet there was no seizure activity. She did, however, suffer from insomnia, sleeping approximately two hours at a time and then staying awake and active for two or three days without a break.

When first seen, she was on multiple seizure medications, including Topamax (as well as Klonopin for sleep and Resperdal for ADHD). The last seizure, however, was 2–2 1/2 years previous. Yet the medications were continued, even though Summer demonstrated a normal sleep EEG. She was also on Carnitor and CoQ 10 for mitochondrial disease and Zantac for GI problems. Although she remained very active and mobile, the main physical problem was still the hypotonia of the hips. She was flat-footed with no arc. Her upper motor coordination was poor, but weight was acceptable for size. Secondary diagnoses included epilepsy, sensory integration deficits, and autistic behavior.

The results following 19 hyperbaric oxygen treatments have thus far been dramatic. Summer can now walk up and down stairs with one hand on the railing, something she had never been able to do before. In fact, she gets annoyed when someone tries to help her (which she absolutely needed before). Now it's, "No, Mom, I do it!" and she runs up and down the stairs. She is learning to feed herself. Her speech is improving, and she is saying meaningful 3–4 word sentences. Cognitive improvements include better understanding and response to commands. Her attentiveness is improving as she learns to use her visual skills and integrate them with her surroundings. She is being taken off the Klonopin at this point. Her basic coordination is greatly enhanced in activities such as pulling string toys and putting blocks in matching holes. Summer, for the first time, has developed not only the ability but the initiative to do things like put her shoes and socks on by herself. The first time, admittedly, it was the right shoe on the left foot, but at least she put the socks on first. Small steps perhaps, but great leaps when you are a Mom.

Brooke

The following is observations of Brooke's history prior to hyperbaric oxygen treatment in her mom's own words:

Brooke was born in April of 1999 via C-section at 32 weeks' gestation, and had a twin brother. Brooke weighed 3.8 pounds at birth and stayed in the hospital three and a half weeks following birth.

Her development was slower than her twin in all areas, but was considered within normal limits by her pediatrician. She had two seizures in one day at age five months. She had another seizure a month later. She had a normal brain MRI in September 1999. Her neurologist followed her for approximately a year and a half. When he dismissed her, he felt she would need no further neurological treatment.

All of Brooke's well-baby check-ups were normal. At her four-year check-up, she was referred to a pediatric ophthalmologist. It was found that she had accommodative esotropia. She was prescribed glasses. She was also given her four-year immunizations (two in the left leg and one in the left arm) at this check-up in May of 2003.

Brooke was very verbal before she became ill; at times we complained that she talked all the time. In the latter part of May, after the vaccines, we noticed that she was drooling more than normal, and her speech, at times, seemed to be strained. An even more dramatic development was that she didn't talk very much anymore. During this time frame, she vomited on several occasions with no apparent illness. She also felt a little warm from time to time, and people would comment that she felt like she had a fever.

Around the middle of June she had a bowel movement in our above ground pool; this was very unusual because she was potty trained at the time. We just assumed this was an accident (but now, we're not so sure). The last four times she got in the pool, she had a BM in her swimsuit. When asked why she did not tell us she had to go, she said, "I was in a hurry," or, "It was an accident." Also, while riding in the car she would suddenly announce, "I wet my panties." I don't think she could control her kidneys and bowel functions at this time.

Later in June, she started really having trouble with her speech. Her twin had gone through two spells of stuttering that were short-lived, so we assumed that's what was going on with Brooke. It was as though she knew what she wanted to say but couldn't get her words out.

One day in July of 2003, she got up and couldn't bend her left leg. She was walking stiff-legged. We panicked and took her to her pediatrician's office. He said he felt some clonus in her left leg/ankle and referred her to a pediatric orthopedist. Her appointment was two weeks later. The only thing we mentioned to him was her walk. We didn't realize the other issues could possibly be related. He looked at her history and told us he thought she had a mild case of cerebral palsy. We were devastated. He referred us to her previous neurologist, but as it was two weeks before she could be seen, we asked for an MRI of the brain so that we could have the results before our appointment. This was done. It was at least four weeks from the time we noticed her awkward gait; her condition was worsening and she was receiving no treatment, however, she did begin physical therapy for CP. It was during this time frame that her hands and arms began to shake when she tried for fine motor control in the act of picking up anything.

On August 21, 2003, we returned to the neurologist. He immediately told us that it was not CP, but that her brain MRI was "very disturbing." He admitted her to Scottish Rite Children's Hospital the next morning. They performed a spinal MRI, spinal tap, and numerous blood tests and had a pediatric ophthalmologist look at her. The neurologist told us that the best-case scenario would be encephalitis, or brain inflammation. He also told us that he could not rule out a metabolic or mitochondrial cause. He informed us that he would treat her with IV steroids for a five-day regimen. He stated that if she responded to the steroids, it would be a good sign, and that hopefully it was only an inflammatory problem. The steroids were started that day. By the next morning, her speech had improved tremendously, and during the course of the steroids she continued to improve. Her neurologist had by then called a geneticist in on the case. She told us that since Brooke had responded to the steroids, she didn't think we needed to do the genetic testing at that time. She told us to call her if Brooke didn't improve. Brooke was released following the five-day steroid treatment and went home on a steroid-weaning schedule.

Back at physical therapy, her therapist was very impressed. She said that Brooke's tone had decreased from 80–90% to 10% and that the clonus was almost gone. Brooke continued to progress, but slowly. Two days after she was completely off the steroids she began regressing. Her gait worsened, as well as her speech and drooling. Now the neurologist stated, "This is not encephalitis." He also said that it was more like a bulbar myelitis. He stated that he did not know what was wrong with her; he had no definite diagnosis. He started her on Prednisalon twice a day: 5 ml in the morning and 5 ml at night. He told us we would wean her off over a ten-week period or so. He said if she continued to progress, great. If not, the next step would be a muscle biopsy. She continued to progress, for awhile.

I had been noticing that her urine was very cloudy, and thought the steroids were probably causing it. I called the doctor's office to see if that could be the case. They told me no, the steroids shouldn't cause it. I was told to bring her in for a urine test. They found white cells and blood in the urine. They sent me home with two samples of the antibiotic Cefzi. They told me they would culture it, but they felt sure she had a urinary tract infection. To everyone's surprise, the culture was negative, so nothing further was done. That afternoon about 1:00 Brooke started complaining of stomach pain. We were on the way to physical therapy, so I guess she was preoccupied and forgot about it. By 4:00 she was doubled over, complaining of pain in her right side. I took her back to the doctor's office. He said her white cells were 12,000 (8,000 is normal). He sent her to the Medical Center of Central Georgia for an abdominal X-ray. Once we got to the hospital she got much worse and vomited five times in an hour time frame. She was very shaky and still doubled over with pain. They did another white cell count and it had skyrocketed to 27,000 (while another test done at 5:00 a.m. the following morning revealed a count of 11,000). She was admitted with appendicitis in mind. At this point, Brooke was very unresponsive to everything and everyone. Surgeons came in and decided that it probably was not appendicitis, but wanted to watch her overnight and order a CAT scan if warranted. It was decided that the CAT scan was not needed. Although they had no diagnosis, appendicitis was ruled out. They did find that she was dehydrated and gave her two bags of fluid. She was better the next day and no further testing was done. They started her on two broad-spectrum IV antibiotics. The urine they collected at the hospital was cloudy. The nurse even commented on it. The nurse told me it had white cells and protein in it. However, the attending doctor said it was fine. The culture was negative. She was released from the hospital about 6:00 p.m. on October 17, again with no diagnosis.

On October 12, just prior to her hospitalization, her therapist had been quite pleased with progress. She then had good balance (for her), and was able to walk the balance beam while holding the therapist's hand. After this latest illness, however, she continued to regress. Her balance worsened to the point that she could not walk without holding on to someone or something. When she took two or three steps on her own, she would veer to the right and could not walk in a straight line.

By now, the shaking of her hands and arms was at times uncontrollable, and she would drop what she was holding. Much of the time she could not even pick up a glass or feed herself because of the shaking.

On the afternoon of October 25, while trying to get her Papa to sleep, after a few minutes of silence she said, "Papa, I can't walk." Her mind is very keen, and she knows exactly what is happening, but she is slow in phrasing her thoughts and responding. However, she is very quick to grasp what is going on. Unlike most four-year-olds, Brooke worried about her condition and all that was happening.

I called and talked to the neurologist (on call) on October 25. I explained most of the above and told him that Brooke will not (or cannot) walk on her own, she has to hold on to something or someone to ambulate, that this was frightening and worse than before. Brooke was once again admitted to the hospital. By this point we were desperate for answers and a diagnosis. Finally, a muscle biopsy was performed, and it appeared to be a mitochondrial disease, most probably Leigh's.

When seen at the Ocean Hyperbaric Neurologic Center in January of 2004, the mother stated that Brooke, now 4 3/4 years old, had continued to deteriorate. She could no longer talk at all. She could no longer walk, turn, or crawl. In appearance, she was a well-developed, well-nourished child, with a slight "moon face" secondary to the cortisone.

She was small and very alert, but was unable to express herself in any way. Both lower extremities were positive for low grade clonus, with slight clonus of the right hand. There was generalized severe weakness of all four extremities. She could not hold her head up nor her torso erect. Baseline SPECT brain scan revealed multiple areas of hypoperfusion and patchiness, indicating decreased blood flow and thereby limited oxygen metabolism (Fig. 4). The patient was begun on hyperbaric oxygen treatments at 1.25 ATA concomitant with all standard modalities of PT, OT, and speech therapy. Following 74 HBO treatments, repeat SPECT scanning demonstrated significant improvement in the cerebral cortical flow (Fig.5). The previous occipital defects had disappeared and these regions were now well perfused.

As of April, 2004, she had received 78 hyperbaric oxygen treatments with dramatic results. Brooke is now back in school. She is walking and feeding herself and continues to improve. Her speech and mentation have improved, and she is now speaking in full sentences and continues to improve cognitively. Brooke now takes steps independently and can bend her knee, neither of which she was able to do prior to the hyperbaric oxygen treatments. Brooke is able to control her bowel/bladder independently and is now consistent with her bowel movements. Emotionally, she is able to giggle and laughs appropriately; in fact, she has quite a sense of humor.

Her parents report that her overall stability is becoming closer to normal, and both her independent neurologist and physician feel that the hyperbaric oxygen played a definite role in her amazing progress.

Conclusion

Explanations for the phenomena herein observed on the admittedly few cases of mitochondrial cytopathies treated with HBO remain somewhat elusive. But the most likely conclusions are that hyperbaric oxygen exerts a positive effect on the mitochondria in their production of ATP; utilization of glucose, amino acids, and oxygen; and cell respiration. HBOT apparently rectifies certain problems in the mitochondrial function by either increasing cytochrome production, altering the structure of proteins, or increasing the efficiency of the cytochromes already present. In all probability it also has the ability to selectively turn mitochondrial genes on and off. The emerging understanding of the mechanisms of HBOT in treating mitochondrial cytopathies is generating new and exciting concepts for the use of the ever-expanding field of hyperbaric oxygenation in the treatment of the brain-injured child.

With more recent scientific evidence in mitochondrial studies and imaging, multiple diseases are now linked to mitochondrial failure not only in children, but also adults in liver, cardiac, renal system, and brain (including Alzheimer's, etc.) Previously mentioned was the recognized effect of carbon monoxide on cytochrome c, but a recent paper in the *Journal of Neurosurgery* (2004) clearly shows the effect of mitochondrial damage in traumatic brain injury in the experimental animal. This parallels the work with hyperbaric oxygen that we have been doing for years in humans and the logic of this approach becomes even clearer.

Mitochondria, however, is its own worst enemy. Organs which require more energy (brain, heart, etc.) have more mitochondria and are more susceptible to its damage. Electron transport, hydroxyl radicals and reactive oxygen species (ROS) are routinely formed as basic mechanisms of the cell, yet they tend to destroy the mytochondria. The body has produced mechanisms to try to defeat this with UPC (uncoupling) enzyme which has recently been found to have been a basic defense in both animal and plants for centuries. When they are released, ROS supercedes mitochondrial function. Mitochondrial failure results in many disease states, and is even found in the basic human aging process. Thus, mitochondrial disorders are not simply limited to inherent genetic diseases in children. This is a whole new field of medical research and this chapter is the first publication to suggest that hyperbaric oxygenation may indeed turn on good genes, turn off bad genes, and positively alter and enhance the function of the mitochondria and production of ATP.

I am indebted to my daughter, Virginia Neubauer, for extrapolating my knowledge and expressing it in understandable terms, and to Sheldon Gottlieb, Ph.D., for his scientific input.

PUBLICATIONS
Materials written for publication by Dr. Richard Neubauer

Neubauer RA. High dose oxygen therapy for mental retardation and developmental delays in children with cerebral palsy. *Proceedings of Mental Retardation in Childhood II*, Lillehammer, Norway. Apr 6-8, 2000.

Neubauer RA. High dose oxygen enhances paediatric neuromuscular rehabilitation. *Proceedings of International Meeting in Paediatric Neuromuscular Rehabilitation*, Coimbra, Portugal. Mar 23-25, 2000.

Neubauer RA. Hyperbaric oxygenation in cerebral palsy and the brain injured child. *Proceedings of the 3rd European Paediatric Neurology Society*, Nice, France. 283-289, Nov 7-10, 1999.

Neubauer RA, Uszler JM, James PB. Hyperbaric oxygenation: the recoverable brain in certain pediatric patients. *Proceedings of 8th International Child Neurology Congress*, Ljubljana, Slovenia. 475-480, Sept 13-18, 1998.

Neubauer RA. Hyperacute hyperbaric oxygen for CNS ischemia. *Proceedings of Interdisciplinary Symposium on Hyperbaric Oxygen Therapy*, Gottingen. 71-76, 1998.

Neubauer RA. Hyperbaric oxygen as an adjunct in strokes due to thrombosis. *Proceedings of Interdisciplinary Symposium on Hyperbaric Oxygen Therapy*, Gottingen. 77-80, 1998.

Neubauer RA, James PB. Cerebral oxyenation and the recoverable brain. *Neuro Res* 20 (Suppl 1) S33-S36, 1998.

Neubauer RA, Gottlieb SF. Long-term anoxic encephalopathy: predictability of recovery. *Proceedings of International Joint Meeting on Hyperbaric and Underwater Medicine*, Milan, Italy. Sept 8, 1996.

Neubauer RA, James PB. Free radicals and antioxidants. Lancet (Ltr.), 344: 1440-1441, Nov 19, 1994.

Neubauer RA, Gottlieb SF. Hyperbaric oxygen in closed head injury. *Southern Med J*, 87(9): 933-936, Sept 1994.

Neubauer RA, Gottlieb SF. Hyperbaric oxygen for brain injury. (Ltr.), *J of Neurosurg*, 78: 687-688, Apr 1993.

Neubauer RA, Gottlieb SF. Hyperbaric oxygen, idling neurons, and stroke management. (Ltr.), *J of Critical Illness*, 8(8), Aug 1993.

Neubauer RA, Gottlieb SF. Results of a prospective randomized trial treatment for severely brain-injured patients with hyperbaric oxygen (Ltr.), *J of Neurosurg* (in press, Apr 1993).

Neubauer RA, Gottlieb SF. Hyperbaric oxygen therapy leading to recovery of a 6-week comatose patient afflicted by anoxic encephalopathy and post-traumatic edema. *J of Hyperbaric Med* (Ltr.), 7(1): 57-61, Mar 1992.

Neubauer RA, Gottlieb SF, Miale A, Jr. Identification of hypometabolic areas in the brain using brain imaging and hyperbaric oxygen. *J Clin Med*, 17(6): 477-482, June 1992.

Neubauer RA, Gottlieb SF. Reversal of a dense, persistent, holohemispheric neurological deficit after an endarterectomy of the carotid artery: case report. *Neurosurg* (Ltr.), 30(2): 301-302, 1992.

Neubauer RA, Gottlieb SF. Radionuclide imaging techniques in the evaluation of HBOT effects. *Proceedings of the XVII Annual Meeting of the European Undersea and Baromedical Society on Diving and Hyperbaric Medicine*, Crete, Greece. 269: Sept 29-Oct 3, 1991.

Neubauer RA, Gottlieb SF. Hyperbaric oxygen therapy in unstable angina. In: Pallotta R (ed) *Proceedings of the World Meeting of Hyperbaric Medicine*. International Society of Hyperbaric Medicine, Naples, 1991 (in press).

Neubauer RA, Gottlieb SF. A theoretical comparison between organic pharmaceuticals and hyperbaric oxygen in the treatment of brain injury. In: *Abstracts from the Proceedings World Meeting of Hyperbaric Medicine. International Society of Hyperbaric Medicine*, Naples, 51-52: 1991.

Neubauer RA, Gottlieb SF, Miale A. Imaging techniques in the evaluation of HBOT effects. In: *Abstracts from the Proceedings World Meeting of Hyperbaric Medicine*. International Society of Hyperbaric Medicine, Naples, 17-18: 1991.

Neubauer RA, Gottlieb SF. Stroke Treatment. *Lancet* (Ltr.), 337: 1601, June 29, 1991.

Neubauer RA, Gottlieb SF, Kagan RL. Enhancing "idling" neurons. *Lancet* (Ltr.), 542: Mar 3,1990.

Neubauer RA. Carbon monoxide intoxication - an insidious CNS problem. In: *Abstracts from the Proceedings: 5th International Congress on Neurotoxicology and Occupational Neurology*, Prague, Czechoslovakia, 10: Sept 24-27, 1990.

Neubauer RA. Severe natural gas poisoning successfully treated with hyperbaric oxygen - 2 years later. In: *Abstracts from the Proceedings: 5th International Congress on Neurotoxicology and Occupational Neurology*, Prague, Czechoslovakia 10: Sept 24-27, 1990.

James PB, Neubauer RA. Hyperbaric oxygen in the management of multiple sclerosis. In: Jain KK (ed) *Textbook of Hyperbaric Medicine*. Hogrefe & Huber, Bern, Switzerland, pp 254-261: 1990.

Hill RK, Jr., Bright DE, Neubauer RA. Use of hyperbaric oxygen in the reanastomosis of the severed ear: a review. *J of Hyperbaric Med*, (4)4: 163-176, 1989.

Neubauer RA, Gottlieb SF. Hyperbaric oxygen for acute carbon monoxide intoxication (letter). *Lancet*, 1989 (in press).

Neubauer RA, Kagan RL, Gottlieb SF, James PB. Delayed metabolism or reperfusion in brain imaging after exposure to hyperbaric oxygenation - a therapeutic indicator? (Poster) *Proceedings of XVth Annual Meeting EUBS 89 on Diving and Hyperbaric Medicine,* Israeli Navy Publications, Haifa, Israel, 358-363: 1989.

Neubauer RA, Kagan RL, Gottlieb SF, James PB. Delayed metabolism, reperfusion or redistribution in iofetamine brain imaging after exposure to hyperbaric oxygen: clinical correlations. *Proceedings of XVth Annual Meeting EUBS 89 on Diving and Hyperbaric Medicine,* Israeli Navy Publications, Haifa, Israel, 237-243: 1989.

Gottlieb SF, James PB, Neubauer RA. The evolving use of HBO in MS. *Proceedings of XVth Annual Meeting EUBS 89 on Diving and Hyperbaric Medicine*, Israeli Navy Publications, Haifa, Israel, 231-236: 1989.

Neubauer RA, Kagan RL, Gottlieb SF, James PB. When is stroke completed? Demonstration of the ischemic penumbra. *Proceedings of XVth Annual Meeting EUBS 89 on Diving and Hyperbaric Medicine*, Israeli Navy Publications, Haifa, Israel, 224-230: 1989.

Gottlieb SF, Neubauer RA, James PB. Is hyperbaric oxygen a viable treatment for MS? *Proceedings 2nd International Congress on Hyperbaric Medicine,* Kos, Greece, September 13-15, 1989.

Neubauer RA, Kagan RL, Gottlieb SF, James PB. Reactivation of the ischemic penumbra, delayed metabolism, or reperfusion in CNS dysfunction following hyperbaric oxygen as demonstrated by SPECT. *Proceedings 2nd International Congress on Hyperbaric Medicine,* Kos, Greece, September 13-15, 1989.

Neubauer RA, Kagan RL, Gottlieb SF, James PB. A potential guide to therapy in CNS dysfunction - SPECT analysis, Iofetamine, hyperbaric oxygen. *Proceedings 2nd International Congress on Hyperbaric Medicine,* Kos, Greece, September 13-15, 1989.

Neubauer RA, Kagan RL, Gottlieb SF. Use of hyperbaric oxygen for the treatment of aseptic bone necrosis: a case study. *J of Hyperbaric Med* 4(2): 69-76, June 1989.

Neubauer RA, Pinella J, Hill RK, Bright DE. The use of hyperbaric oxygen in the successful reanastomosis of the severed ear: three cases. (In press) *Proceedings Annual Meeting, European Undersea Biomedical Society,* Aberdeen, Scotland, Sept 5-9, 1988.

Neubauer RA. Hyperbaric oxygen in neurology. Presented at: Inaugural meeting of the International Society of Hyperbaric Medicine, University of Oxford, Sept 1-3, 1988.

Neubauer RA, Kagan RL, Gottlieb SF. Hyperbaric oxygen therapy of aseptic bone necrosis: a case study. (In press) *Proceedings Annual Meeting, European Undersea Biomedical Society,* Aberdeen, Scotland, Sept 5-9, 1988.

Neubauer RA, James PB, Gottlieb SF. HBO Rx multiple sclerosis - A viable therapy? *Proceedings 1988 Undersea and Hyperbaric Medical Society.*

Neubauer RA. Hyperbaric oxygen therapy for multiple sclerosis (Ltr.), *Brit J of Neur, Neurosurg & Psychiatry,* Mar 1988.

Neubauer RA. Smoke inhalation injury. (Ltr.), *Postgraduate Medicine,* Jan 1988.

Neubauer RA, Kagan RL. Alterations in nuclear magnetic imaging (NMI) in multiple sclerosis patients after hyperbaric oxygen treatment. *Proceedings: 11th Ann Conf. Clin. Appl. of Hyperbaric Oxygen,* Long Beach, CA, 54; June 9-13, 1986.

Neubauer RA, Kagan RL. Pitfalls in the use of magnetic resonance imaging (MRI) to evaluate the efficacy of hyperbaric oxygen (HBO) treatment in patients with multiple sclerosis (MS). *Proceedings: 11th Ann Conf. Clin. Appl. of Hyperbaric Oxygen,* Long Beach, CA, 49; June 9-13, 1986.

Neubauer RA. The effect of hyperbaric oxygen in prolonged coma. Possible identification of marginally functioning brain zones. *Medicini Subacquea ed Iperbarica, Edizioni Minerva Medica* 5(3): 75-79; Sept-Dec 1985.

Neubauer RA. Hyperbaric oxygen and multiple sclerosis (letter). *Lancet* 810: Apr 6, 1985.

Neubauer RA. Hyperbaric oxygen therapy of multiple sclerosis. *Medicini Subacquea ed Iperbarica, Edizioni Minerva Med* 3(2) 79-87, 1984.

Neubauer RA, Maxfield JR. Non-union fracture treated 33 months after injury with hyperbaric oxygen. *Medicini Subacquea ed Iperbarica, Edizioni Minerva Medica* 4(1): 23-26; June-Apr, 1984.

Neubauer RA. Protocols for hyperbaric oxygen in multiple sclerosis (letter). *Brit Med J* 288:1831-1832, June 16, 1984.

Neubauer RA. HBO an open letter to all baromedical physicians. *Pressure* 13(1); Feb 1984.

Neubauer RA. Exposure of multiple sclerosis patients to hyperbaric oxygen at 1.5 - 2 ATA: a preliminary report. *J Fla Med Assn* 67:498-504, 1980.

Neubauer RA. Generalized small-vessel stenosis in the brain. A case history of a patient treated with monoplace hyperbaric oxygen at 1.5 to 2 ATA. *Medicini Subacquea ed Iperbarica, Edizioni Minerva Med* 74(35): 2051-5; Sept 15, 1983.

Neubauer RA. A summary of worldwide experience in the treatment of multiple sclerosis with hyperbaric oxygen. In: (Programs and Abstracts) *First Europ. Conf. Hyperbaric Med.* Amsterdam, The Netherlands, 36; Sept 7-9, 1983.

Neubauer RA. Call for clinical trials of HBO (letter). *Med Trib.* 23(20): 23; Sep 29, 1982.

Neubauer RA. Hyperbaric oxygen treatment and stroke (letter). *JAMA* 246(22): 2574; Dec 4, 1981.

Neubauer RA, End E. Hyperbaric oxygenation as an adjunct therapy in strokes due to thrombosis. A review of 122 patients. *Stroke.* 11(3): 297-300; May-Jun 1980.

Neubauer RA. Exposure of multiple sclerosis patients to hyperbaric oxygen at 1.5 - 2 ATA. *J Fla Med Assn* 67: 498-505; (May) 1980.

Neubauer RA. Carbon Monoxide and hyperbaric oxygen (letter). *Arch Intern Med.* 139(7): 829; Jul 1979.

Neubauer RA, End E. Hyperbaric oxygen (editorial). *Am Family Physician.* 19(3): 92-4; Mar 1979.

Neubauer RA. Baromedicine (letter). *MD Med Newsmag.* 22: 24; Sept 1978.

Neubauer RA. Treatment of multiple sclerosis with monoplace hyperbaric oxygen. *J Fla Med Assn* 65:101, 1978.

End E, Neubauer RA. Hyperbaric oxygenation (letter). *Am Family Physician.* 18(2): 23,26; Aug 1978.

Neubauer RA. Common misconceptions about hyperbaric oxygen. *Med Tribune.* 19(18): 7-8; May 10, 1978.

Neubauer RA. Hyperbaric oxygen and leg ulcers (letter). *JAMA.* 239(14): 1393; Apr 3, 1978.

Neubauer RA, End E. Scuba diving with MS. *Physician and Sportsmed.* 6: 13; Feb 1978.

PRESENTATIONS

Presented by Dr. Richard Neubauer at major international conferences

2001
New Hope for the Neurologically Damaged Child, Cerebral Palsy, Anoxic Ischemic Encephalopathy, and Traumatic Brain Injury
> "What is hyperbaric oxygen therapy? How is it administered? What are its effects in children with cerebral palsy and brain injury?"
> "Hyperbaric Oxygenation—An Overview"

2000
New Integrative Medicine Treatments for Cancer and Chronic Illnesses
Anaheim, California   November 11, 2000
> "Hyperbaric oxygen treatments in integrative medicine"

5th Congress of the European Federation of Neurological Societies
Copenhagen, Denmark   October 14 – 18, 2000
> "High dose oxygen therapy in stroke"

26th Annual Meeting of the European Underwater and Baromedical Society on Diving and Hyperbaric Medicine
Malta   September 14 – 17, 2000
> "High dose oxygen therapy in cerebral palsy and the brain injured child"
> "Sequential SPECT imaging / hyperbaric oxygenation in long-term neurologic deficits."
> "Hyperbaric oxygenation in acute stroke - 4 hour window"
> "Hyperbaric oxygenation for Lyme Vasculitis"

24th Annual Williamsburg Traumatic Brain Injury Rehabilitation Conference
Williamsburg, VA   June 2 – 4, 2000
> "Hyperbaric oxygenation for cerebral palsy and the brain injured child"

Proceedings of Mental Retardation in Childhood II
Norway   April 6 – 8, 2000
> "High dose oxygen therapy for mental retardation and developmental delays in children with cerebral palsy"

7th Annual Meeting of the American Society of Neurorehabilitation
San Diego, CA   April 27 – 29, 2000
  "Supplemental high dose oxygen therapy facilities neuro-rehabilitation"

Proceedings of International Meeting in Paediatric Neuromuscular Rehabilitation
Coimbra, Portugal   March 23 – 25, 2000
  "High dose oxygen enhances paediatric neuromuscular rehabilitation"

Proceedings of Neuronal Plasticity
Kananaskis, Alberta, Canada   March 19 – 22, 2000
  "The Key to Stroke Recovery"

1999
Proceedings of the 3rd European Paediatric Neurology Society
Nice, France   November 7 – 10, 1999

13th International Congress on Hyperbaric Medicine
Kobe, Japan   November 7 – 12, 1999
  "World Federation of Neurology proposed pilot study of hyperbaric oxygen treatment of acute ischemic thrombotic stroke"
  "Hyperbaric oxygenation for cerebral palsy and the brain injured child"

Coast Chapter of the Undersea and Hyperbaric Medical Society 1999 Scientific Meeting
Marietta, Georgia   October 21 – 23, 1999
  "The use of hyperbaric oxygenation in the hyperacute ischemic thrombotic stroke (WFN proposed pilot study)"
  "Visualization and reactivation of the recoverable brain SPECT/HBO"

4th Congress of the European Federation of Neurologic Societies
Lisbon, Portugal   September 7 – 11, 1999
  "Co-Sponsor – Special Workshop"
  "Introduction to hyperbaric treatments"

1998
Proceedings of 8th International Child Neurology Congress
Ljubjana, Slovenia   September 13 – 18, 1998
  "Hyperbaric oxygenation: the recoverable brain in certain pediatric patients" (with PB James and JM Uszler)

5th International Conference on Functional Mapping of the Human Brain
Dusseldorf, Germany   June 23 – 26, 1998
  "Brain mapping of the injured brain: SPECT/hyperbaric oxygenation"

Congress on Cerebral Ischemia, Vascular Dementia, Epilepsy and CNS Injury, World Federation of Neurology
Washington, D.C.   May 9 – 13, 1998
  "Hyperbaric oxygen therapy in hyper-acute stroke"

1996

Proceedings of International Meeting on Hyperbaric and Underwater Medicine
Milan, Italy   September 8, 1996
  "Long-term anoxic encephalopathy: predictability of recovery"
  (With SF Gottlieb)

2nd Annual Conference on Functional Mapping of the Human Brain
Boston, MA   June 17 – 21, l996
  "Brain mapping in anoxic encephalopathy – SPECT / hyperbaric oxygenation"

Annual Meeting of the Southeastern Chapter of the Society of Nuclear Medicine
Atlanta, GA   1996
  "Visualization of reperfusion and/or recoverable brain" (With NH Pevsner)

XXII Annual Meeting of the European Underwater Baromedical Society, XII International Congress on Hyperbaric Medicine, III Consensus Conference of the ECHM Joint Meeting
Milano, Italy   September 4 – 8, l996
  "Sequential SPECT scanning in long term anoxic encephalopathy"

20th Annual Postgraduate Course on Rehabilitation of the Brain Injured Adult & Child
Williamsburg, VA   June 6 – 9, 1996
  "Brain Challenge – SPECT/HBO – long-term closed head injury"

1995

Undersea and Hyperbaric Medical Society, Gulf Coast Chapter Annual Scientific Assembly
New Orleans, LA   March 30 – April 2, 1995
  "Prognosis in early stroke: SPECT scanning"

Gulf Coast Chapter Annual Scientific Assembly. Undersea and Hyperbaric Medical Society
San Antonio, TX   March 21 – 24, 1995
  "Brain Challenge – SPECT / hyperbaric oxygen" (With SF Gottlieb)

1992

1992 Undersea and Hyperbaric Medical Society Annual Scientific Meeting
Bethesda, MD   June 23 – 27, l992
  "Amelioration of long term head injuries with hyperbaric oxygen – documentation via SPECT brain imaging" (Poster) (With SF Gottlieb)

1992 Gulf Coast Chapter Undersea and Hyperbaric Medical Society Annual Scientific Meeting
San Antonio, TX   March 26 – 29, 1992
  "Interventional brain imaging; identification of idling neurons with hyperbaric documentation via SPECT brain imaging" (Poster)

1991
PanEuropean Society of Neurology Second Congress
Vienna, Austria   December 8 – 14, l991
"Is there recoverable brain tissue in closed head injury? SPECT imaging, HBOT and clinical correlation"

Proceedings of the XVII Annual Meeting of the European Undersea and Baromedical Society on Diving and Hyperbaric Medicine
Crete, Greece   September 29 – October 3, 1991
"Radionuclide imaging techniques in the evaluation of HBOT effects" (With SF Gottlieb)

International Society of Hyperbaric Medicine
Naples   1991
Abstract from the Proceedings:
"Imaging techniques in the evaluation of HBOT effects"
"A theoretical comparison between organic pharmaceuticals and hyperbaric oxygen in the treatment of brain injuries" (With SF Gottlieb)

First Hispano-American Meeting on Diving and Hyperbaric Medicine
Havana, Cuba   July 7 – 14, 1991
"Anoxic/hyoxic encephalopathies"
"Overall use of HBO in neurologic diseases"
"HBO in acute and chronic deficit of stroke"
"Multiple sclerosis. Long term evaluation"
"Metabolic imagining: the ischemic penumbra"
"Neurologic applications of hyperbaric oxygen in closed head injury, vegetative coma, and anoxic encephalopathies"

1990
IX Scientific Meeting of the Italian Society of Underwater and Hyperbaric Medicine
Lerici, Italy   September 28 – 30, 1990
"Varying pictures of stoke"
"MS revisited: The truth emerges"
"Hyperbaric oxygen – central nervous system" (With SF Gottlieb)

5th International Congress on Neurotoxicology and Occupational Neurology
Prague, Czechoslovakia   September 24 – 27, 1990
"Carbon monoxide intoxication – an insidious CNS problem" (Abstract)
"Severe natural gas poisoning successfully treated with hyperbaric oxygen – 2 years later" (Abstract)

1990 Joint Meeting on Diving and Hyperbaric Medicine – International Congress on Hyperbaric Medicine (Undersea and Hyperbaric Medical Society and European Undersea Biomedical Society)
Amsterdam, The Netherlands   August 11 – 18, 1990
"Visibility of ischemic penumbra demonstrated by SPECT/HBO" (With FS Gottlieb)

1989

Proceedings of XVth Annual Meeting EUBS 89 on Diving and Hyperbaric Medicine
Haifa, Israel   1989
"Delayed metabolism or reperfusion in brain imaging after exposure to
hyperbaric oxygenation – a therapeutic indicator?"
"Delayed metabolism, reperfusion or redistribution in iofetamine brain
imaging after exposure to hyperbaric oxygen: clinical correlations"
"The evolving use of HBO in MS"
"When is stroke completed? Demonstration of the ischemic penumbra"
(With RL Kagan, SF Gottlieb, and PB James)

Proceedings 3nd International Congress on Hyperbaric Medicine
Kos, Greece   September 13 – 15, 1989
"A potential guide to therapy in CNS dysfunction – SPECT analysis,
iofetamine, hyperbaric oxygen"
"Is hyperbaric oxygen a viable treatment for MS?"
"When is stroke completed? Demonstration of the ischemic penumbra"
"Reactivation of the ischemic penumbra, oxygen as demonstrated by
SPECT" (With RL Kagan, SF Gottlieb, and PB James)

**Proceedings, 1989 Undersea and Hyperbaric Medical Society Annual Scientific
Meeting**
Honolulu, Hawaii   June 7 – 11, 1989
"The use of hyperbaric oxygen for the treatment of aseptic bone narcosis: a
case study"
"Improved metabolism in marginal brain tissue by hyperbaric oxygen (HBO)
as visualized by I-123 Iofetamine analysis" (With RL Kagan and SF Gottlieb)

First International Conference of Bio-Oxidative Medicine
Dallas, Texas   February 17 – 20, 1989
"Tissue healing and regeneration augmented by hyperbaric oxygen therapy"

Annual Meeting, European Undersea Biomedical Society
Aberdeen, Scotland   September 5 – 9, 1989
"Hyperbaric oxygen therapy of aseptic bone necrosis: a case study"
(With RA Kagan, and SF Gottlieb)
"The use of hyperbaric oxygen in the successful reanastomosis
of the severed ear: three cases"
(With J Pinella, RK Hill, and DE Bright)

Inaugural Meeting of the International Society of Hyperbaric Medicine
University of Oxford   September 1 – 3, 1989
"Hyperbaric oxygen in neurology"

1988

1988 Undersea and Hyperbaric Medical Society (Proceedings)
"HBO Rx multiple sclerosis – A viable therapy?"
(With PB James and SF Gottlieb)

1st Beinalle Del Mar, International Meeting of Diving and Hyperbaric Medicine
Naples, Italy   June 5 – 12, 1988
"Neuroimmunologic and neurologic indications for hyperbaric oxygen"

1987

XIIIth Annual Meeting of the European Undersea Biomedical Society
Palermo, Italy   September 9 – 12, 1987
"Positive effects of hyperbaric oxygen in multiple sclerosis—double-blind and longitudinal data" (With SF Gottlieb)

1987 Spring Conference American College of Advancement in Medicine
Orlando, FL   May 7 – 10, 1987
"Hyperbaric oxygen in certain function preservation and tissue repair"

Annual Meeting Gulf Coast Chapter UHMS
April 1987
"A reappraisal positive effects of hyperbaric oxygen in multiple sclerosis – double-blind and longitudinal data" (With SF Gottlieb)

1987 Annual UMS/Gulf Coast Chapter Meeting
Orlando, FL   March 20 – 21, 1987
"Current aspects of multiple sclerosis and hyperbaric oxygen I and II" (With SF Gottlieb)

1986

First Annual Hyperbaric Medical Symposium of Hyperbaric Medicine
Basle, Switzerland   October 14 – 15, 1986
"Hyperbaric oxygen therapy of vegetative coma patients"
"Hyperbaric oxygen therapy of stroke"
"A critique of recent studies in hyperbaric oxygen and multiple sclerosis" (With PB James and SF Gottlieb)
"Magnetic resonance imaging and evoked potential recordings in multiple sclerosis patients using hyperbaric oxygen therapy"

11th Annual Conference of Clinical Applications in Hyperbaric Oxygen and Multiple Sclerosis Patients (Proceedings)
Long Beach, CA   June 9 – 13, 1986
"Pitfalls in the use of magnetic resonance imaging (MRI) to evaluate the efficacy of hyperbaric oxygen (HBO) treatment in patients with multiple sclerosis (MS)" (With RL Kagan)
"Alterations in nuclear magnetic imaging (NMI) in multiple sclerosis patients after hyperbaric oxygen treatment" (With RL Kagan)
"Hyperbaric oxygen therapy of stroke" (With RL Kagan)

1985
III World Congress of Neurology
Hamburg, Germany   September 1 – 6, 1985
> "Changes in the magnetic resonance imaging after hyperbaric oxygen treatment in multiple sclerosis patients" (With MA Morariu)
> "Somatosensory evoked potentials before and after hyperbaric medicine treatment in patients with multiple sclerosis" (With MA Morariu)

X Congress EUBS
Marseille, France   1985
> "The effect of hyperbaric oxygen therapy in multiple sclerosis as evaluated by nuclear magnetic resonance"

International Symposium on HBO in Critical Care Medicine
Eliat, Israel   June 30 – July 3, 1985
> "The treatment of focal edema in the central nervous system by hyperbaric oxygen demonstrated by magnetic resonance imaging" (With PB James)

1984
International Meeting of HBO
Long Beach, CA   August 1984
> "rCBF studies before and after diseases including stroke and vegetative coma" (With JE Gelety and RJ Centrone)

IX Conference on Clinical Applications of Hyperbaric Oxygen
Acapulco, Mexico   1984
> "The effects of hyperbaric oxygen on evoked potentials in multiple sclerosis patients" (With A Morariu)

Xth Congress of EUBS
Marseille, France   1984
> "Hyperbaric oxygen on magnetic resonance imaging in multiple sclerosis"

1983
First European Conference on Hyperbaric Medicine
Amsterdam, The Netherlands   September 7 – 9, 1983
> "A summary of worldwide experience in the treatment of multiple sclerosis with hyperbaric oxygen"

Eighth Conference on Clinical Applications of Hyperbaric Oxygen
Long Beach, CA   June 1983
> "Long term effects of hyperbaric oxygen in multiple sclerosis"

1982
Congresso Nazionale Meicina Subacquea a Iperbaric
Montecatina   October 1982
> Keynote Address: "Hyperbaric oxygen in neurologic disorders"

Seventh Annual Conference on Clinical Applications of HBO
Anaheim, CA   June 1982
   "Regional cerebral blood flow studies of the effect of hyperbaric oxygen in
   acute stroke and chronic neurological defects of stroke; 30 cases"

1980
5th Annual Conference on Clinical Applications of Hyperbaric Oxygen
Long Beach, CA   June l980
   "rCBF studies before and after hyperbaric oxygen in neurological
   dysfunction using Xenon 133" (With JE Gelety and RJ Centrone)

Gulfstream Chapter Meeting Undersea Medical Society
Houston, TX   March 1980
   "Hyperbaric oxygen therapy in stroke" (With MR Kuhn)

1979
Fourth Annual Conference of Clinical Applications of HBO
Long Beach, CA   l979
   "Treatment of organic brain syndrome with hyperbaric oxygen"
   (With Edgar End)
   "Treatment of multiple sclerosis with monoplace hyperbaric oxygen"
   (With R Schnell and GS Goldberg)

REFERENCES

Behnke AR, Johnson FS, et al. "The Effects of Oxygen on Man." 1935. *American Journal of Physiology.* 110:565 - 572

Beylin GE, Tanapat P, Shors TJ. "Learning enhances adult neurogenesis in the hippocampal formation." 1999. *Nature Neuroscience.* 2:(3) 266.

Boerema I, Meyer NG, et al. "Life without Blood." 1960. *Journal of Cardiovascular Surgery.* 1:133 - 46.

Collet JP, et al. "Hyperbaric Oxygen Therapy in the Treatment of Spastic Diplega Cerebral Palsy." McGill University Pilot Study. 2000. *HBO Today.* (3) 44 - 45.

Collet JP, Vanasse M, Marois P, et al. "Hyperbaric oxygen for children with cerebral palsy: a randomized multicentre trial." 2001. *The Lancet.* 357:582 - 586.

Collet JP, et al. *The Lancet.* Op. cit. 357:586 - 587.

David JC, Hunt TK. Editors. *Hyperbaric Oxygen Therapy.* 1977. UHMS, Bethesda, MD. pp. 3 - 10.

End E, Neubauer RA. "Hyperbaric Oxygenation as an Adjunct Therapy." 1980. *Stroke.* 11:(3) 297 - 300.

Fife CE, Piant A, Dosi C. "Problems in Respiratory Care." 1991. *Hyperbaric Effects of Hyperbaric Hypoxia.* Moon-Editor. J.P. Lippincott, Philadelphia, PA. pp. 150 - 171.

Health Digest. "Study Proves HBO is not Effective." 2001. *Long Beach Press Telegram.* p. 2.

Heuss WD, Graf R. "The Ischemic Penumbra." 1994. *Current Opinions in Neurology.* (US) 7:(1) 11 - 19.

Holback KH, Wassmann H. "Continuous rCBF measurements during hyperbaric oxygen." 1977. *Proceedings of the 6th International Congress on Hyperbaric Medicine.* Aberdeen Universal Press. pp. 104 - 111.

Hunt GB, Kindwall EP. "Hyperbaric Chamber Clinical Support: Monoplace." In: *Hyperbaric Oxygen Therapy.* Davis JC, Hunt TK, (eds.) 1977. Undersea Medical Society, Bethesda, MD. pp. 41 - 46.

Hutchinson J, Kerr M, et al. "Hyperbaric Oxygen in Resuscitation of the Newborn." 1963. *The Lancet.* Vol. 2. pp. 1020 - 1022.

Jain KK. *Textbook of Hyperbaric Medicine*, Third Edition. 1999. Hogrefe & Huber Publishers, Seattle, WA. pp. 17 - 21.

James P. "A Tragic Mistake." 1999. Monduzzi Editore.

James P. "Hyperbaric Oxygen Therapy for Cerebral Palsy Children." 1st International Symposium on Cerebral Palsy and the Brain Injured Child. July 1999. Boca Raton, FL.

Kindwall EP, Whelan HT. Editors. *Hyperbaric Medicine Practice.* 1999. Best Publishing Company, Flagstaff, AZ.

Lambertsen CJ. "Medical Applications of High Oxygen Pressure." 1977. *Transstudy College.* Philadelphia, PA. pp. 1 - 18.

Machado JJ. "Reduction of spasticity clinically observed in patients with neurological disorders, especially children with cerebral palsy." 1989. *Medicine Hyperbarica.* Centro Brasileiro de San Palo, Brazil.

Marois P. Press conference in Quebec. 2001.

McDonald AD. "Oxygen treatment of premature babies and cerebral palsy." 1964. *Develop. Med. Child Neurology.* 6:313 - 314.

Miller F, Bachrach A. *Cerebral Palsy.* 1995. Johns Hopkins Universal Press, Baltimore, MD. pp. 3 - 6.

National Institute of Disabilities and Strokes (NINDS). "Know Your Brain." 1997. U.S. Government Printing Office.

Neubauer RA. "High Dose Oxygen: A Favorable Outcome in Cerebral Palsy and the Brain Injured Child." 2001. Bled, Slovenia.

Neubauer RA. "Hyperbaric oxygenation in cerebral palsy and the brain injured child." *Proceedings of the 3rd EPSN Congress.* 1999. Monduzzi Editors: 283 - 289. Presented at the European Paediatric Neurology Society. November 1999. Nice, France.

Neubauer RA, Gottlieb SF, Kagan RL. "Enhancing 'idling' neurons." 1990. *The Lancet.* (Ltr.) 335:542.

Neubauer RA, Hall-Dickson M. "New Hope." 2000. *Alternative Medicine.* pp. 44 - 49.

Neubauer RA, James P. "Cerebral Oxygenation and the Recoverable Brain." *Neurological Research.* 1998. Vol. 20. Supplement 1.

Neubauer RA, Walker. *Hyperbaric Oxygen Therapy.* 1998. Avery, New York City. pp. 8 - 9.

Neubauer RA, et al. "HBO Treatment for Closed Head Injury." 1994. *Southern Medical Journal.* Vol. 87. No. 9. pp. 933 - 936.

Qibaow W, Hongjun W, Linzheng C, Cuiyun Z. "Treatment of Children's Epilepsy by Hyperbaric Oxygenation: Analysis of 100 Cases." 1995. *Proceedings of the 11th International Congress on Hyperbaric Medicine.* Best Publishing Company, Flagstaff, AZ. pp. 79-81.

Rockswold GL, Ford SF, Anderson DC, et al. "Results of a prospective randomized trial for treatment of severely brain-injured patients with hyperbaric oxygen." 1992. *J Neurosurg.* 76:929 - 934.

Sparacia B. "Diving and Hyperbaric Medicine." 1995. *EUBS 1995 Proceedings.* Helsinki, Finland. pp. 126 - 132.

Sparacia B. "HBO and Brain Injury." 1995. *Min Anest.* Vol. 61. Supp. 2. p. 388.

Trimble V. *The Uncertain Miracle.* 1974. Doubleday, Garden City, NY.

Uszler V. "Video on HBO and Cerebral Palsy." 2001. Produced by Ocean Hyperbaric Center. Lauderdale-by-the-Sea, FL.

Van Heertum BL, Tikofsky RS. Editors. *Functional Cerebral SPECT and PET Imaging.* 1999. J.P. Lippincott, Philadelphia, PA. pp. 1 - 15.

Workman WT. *Hyperbaric Facility Safety: A Practical Guide.* 1999. Best Publishing Company, Flagstaff, AZ. pp. 3 - 8.

Internet Sources

NINDS. "Cerebral Palsy: Hope Through Research." April 21, 2001. 37 pages. From: NINDS website.
www.ninds.nih.gov/health and medica.../cerebral palsy_palsyntr,ht.

Sparacia A. "HBO in the treatment of delayed fetal growth: recent advances in anasth., pain, int., care & emergency." 210 - 218. March 9, 2001. From: webserver of the Institute of Anesthesiology, University of Palermo, Italy.
http://www.unipa.it/care/hbo/fetalgrw.htm.

Steenblock D. "A Brief Review of Hyperbaric Oxygen." November 5, 2000.
www.strokedoctor.com/ story/htm.

Websites

http://member.aol.com/shellic/private/cp.htm

www.hyperbaric.forum.com/ubb/forum56/HTML/0000001.html

www.nimh.nih.gov/sciac/vances/02.cfm

www.torontohyperbaric.com (hyperbaric information resources)

ADDITIONAL REFERENCE MATERIALS

Behnke AR. "A Brief History of Hyperbaric Medicine." In: Davis JC, Hunt TK. *HBOT*. 1977. Underseas Medical Society, Inc. Bethesda, MD. Vol. 8.

Dorland WAN. Editor. *Dorland's Illustrated Medical Dictionary*. 28th edition. 1994. W.B. Saunders, London.

Gerald E, Karn T. *Children with Cerebral Palsy*. 1995. Woodbine House. Philadelphia, PA.

Lambertsen CJ. "Medical Implications of High Oxygen Pressure." *Transstudy College Physicians*. July 1965.

Oberman JP. Lt US Navy Medical Corp. Undersea and Diving Medical Officer. US Navy Report. 1999.

Penderson RA. "Stem Cells for Medicine." *Scientific America*. April 2001.

Rockswold GL, Ford SE, et al. "Treatment of severely injured brain injured patients with hyperbaric oxygen." 1994. *Journal of Neurosurgery*. 76. pp. 929 - 934.